WEIGHT WATCHING SMARTPOINTS

100 + Effective & Delicious WW Smart Points Recipes for Healthy Cooking to Support Your Weight Loss Journey | Includes 30-Day Meal Plan

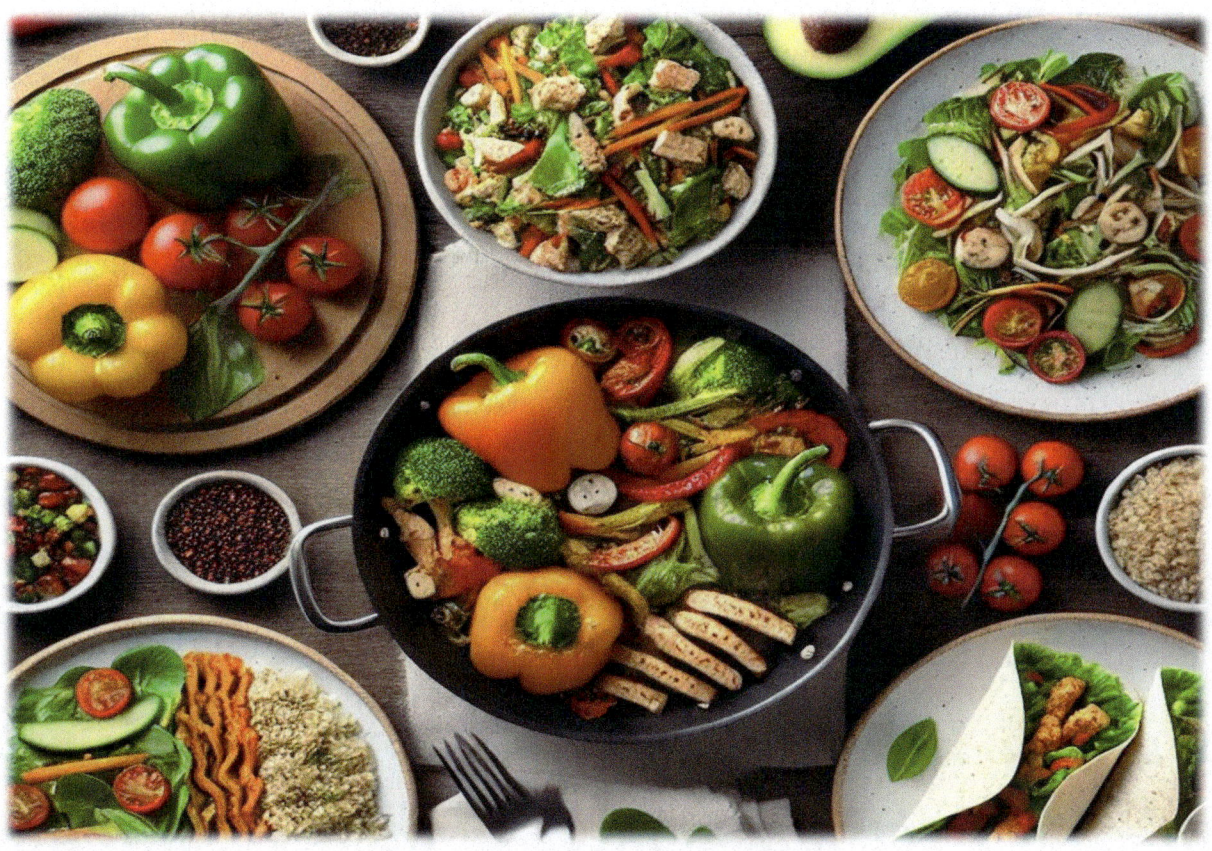

T NISHA

COPYRIGHT © 2025 BY T NISHA

All rights reserved.

This publication permits permitted copyright law brief quotations for critical reviews and noncommercial usages while the publisher alone provides written permission for reproduction, transmission, or distribution through any form or method including photocopying, recording, and electronic or mechanical means.

DISCLAIMER

In the Weight Watching SmartPoints Cookbook for Beginners, the provided recipes serve as general informational material and educational content. The book author together with the publisher declines responsibility for negative impacts that may emerge due to recipe usage in this publication. Before making notable dietary and lifestyle modifications consult with qualified healthcare professionals and nutritionists.

The author and publisher along with other contributors have diligently verified all content but they do not make any promises about what results will occur through following this book's recipes or dietary plans. For average results consult the estimates which use standard measuring standards for ingredients. This book was written to supplement medical information from professional healthcare providers. Talk to medical professionals and qualified dietitians or nutritionists before incorporating new diets and weight loss programs or changing your eating behavior particularly when you have health problems or nutritional restrictions.

The author and the publisher disclaim responsibility for any mistakes in the book's content or for actions taken because of using the provided information.

"With the help of this Book, people take on the Roles of Decision-makers in their Health and Happiness on the WEIGHT WATCHING Journey"

TABLE OF CONTENTS

INTRODUCTION	
Unlocking the Power of the WW SmartPoints System	6
Why SmartPoints Are Key to a Balanced, Healthier Life	9
Setting Yourself Up for Success: A Guide to Starting Strong	10
UNDERSTANDING SMARTPOINTS	
Demystifying SmartPoints: What You Need to Know	11
The Science Behind SmartPoints: How They're Calculated	12
Using SmartPoints to Achieve Long-Term Wellness	13
MASTERING YOUR SMARTPOINTS KITCHEN	
Essential Tools Every WW Kitchen Should Have	14
Stocking Your Pantry with SmartPoints-Friendly Staples	15
Smart Shopping: How to Make Healthier Choices	15
Smart Prep: Time-Saving Tips for Meal Planning and Cooking	16
BREAKFAST DELIGHTS	17
SATISFYING SNACKS AND APPETIZERS	24
HEARTY SOUPS AND STEWS	31
FLAVORFUL SALADS	40
SEAFOOD	48
HEALTHY PLANT-BASED OPTIONS	56
LUNCH IDEAS	64
DELICIOUS DESSERTS	71
SMARTPOINTS COOKING TIPS AND TRICKS	
Cooking with SmartPoints: Tips for Success	78
Simple Techniques to Lower Points Without Sacrificing Flavor	79
EMBRACING A SUSTAINABLE WW LIFESTYLE	
Making WW a Part of Your Everyday Life	80
Practical Strategies for Long-Term Health and Well-being	81
BONUS: 30-DAY MEAL PLAN	82

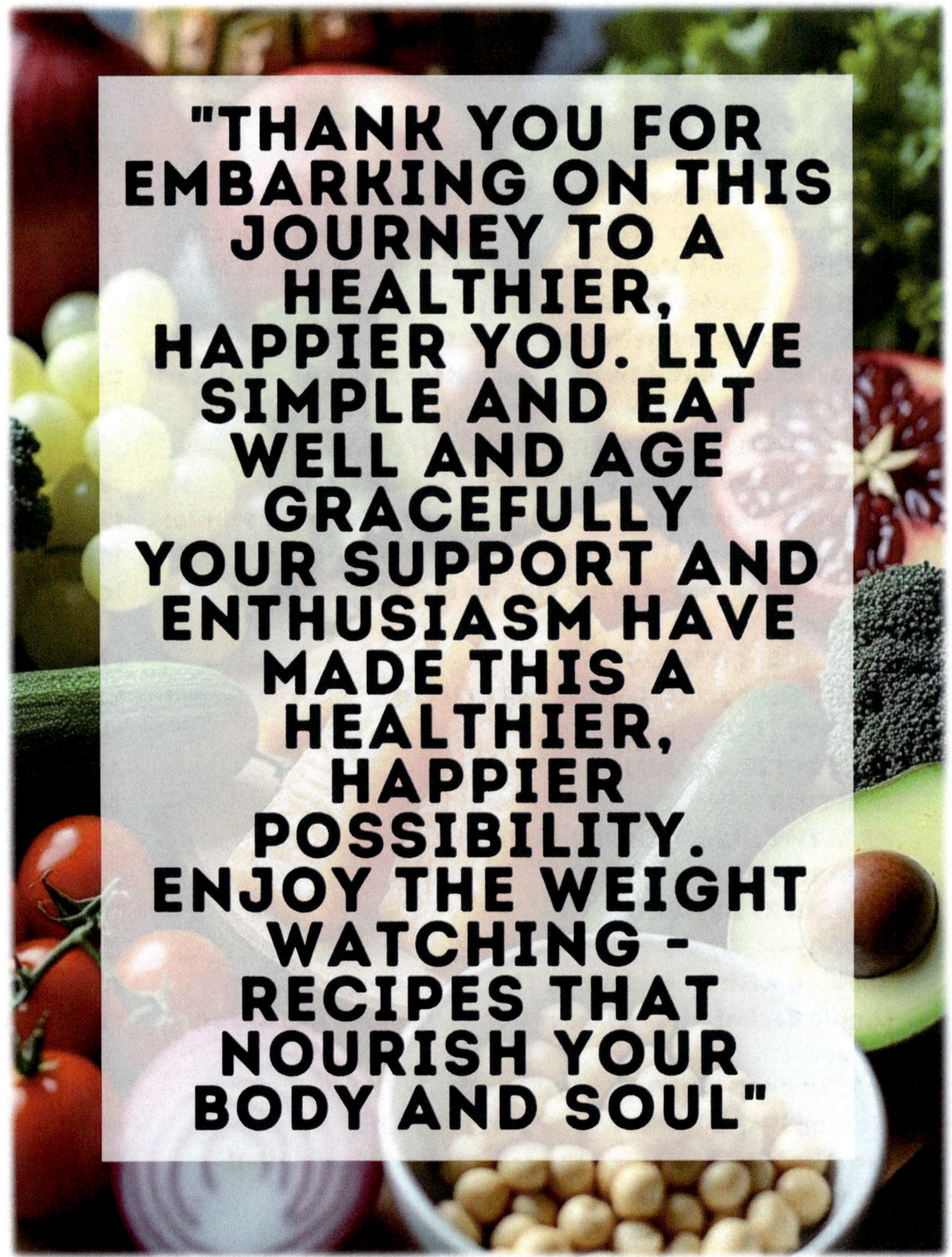

INTRODUCTION

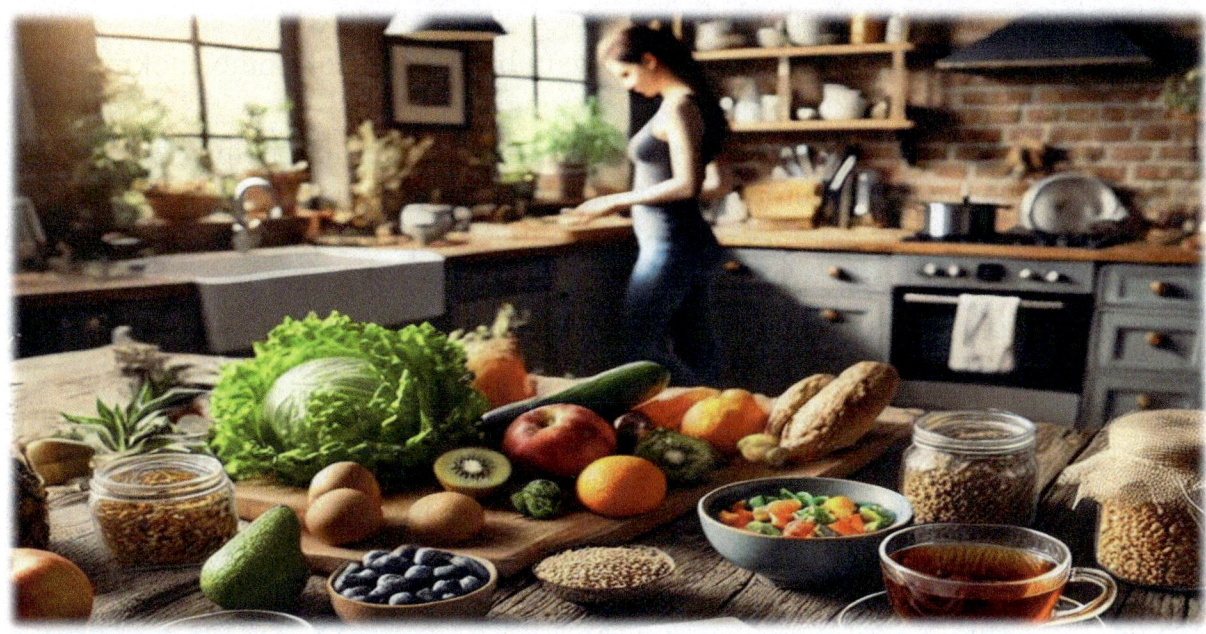

Your life could bring you tasty satisfying food alongside natural weight loss and daily improvement in health status. Sounds too good to be true? It's not. I would like to let you know that the path to reaching your ideal weight marks a departure from food deprivation, an all-foods-off-limits approach, and long cooking sessions in the kitchen. You can build a healthier food relationship and derive pleasure from SmartPoints individually. The Weight Watching SmartPoints Cookbook for Beginners provides this attractive guarantee to its users. This book functions as your essential handbook for healthy cooking and lasting weight loss support for both beginners of the WW (Weight Watchers) program and anyone seeking new simple recipes.

I want to take this opportunity to share an informative tale. Being a mother to two children has left Ana fighting weight problems for many years. She attempted various diets which included low-carb and keto as well as juice cleanse but none of them worked well enough for her. Her state of mind became filled with defeat and overwhelming feelings together with deep frustration. She came across the WW SmartPoints system after that. The plan provided more than meal restriction because it functioned as an entire way of living. Through the WW SmartPoints system, she discovered how to eat healthily while maintaining great taste and enjoyable eating. Six months forward Ana earned multiple achievements by losing 25 pounds along with gaining confidence while feeling more energetic and developing a passion for cooking.

- More than 100 mouth-watering recipes cover the whole day with hearty breakfasts through indulgent dinners and dessert options which are simple to prepare along with their SmartPoints consideration.
- You can succeed in your weight loss journey through a 30-Day Meal Plan which organizes your meals for guided success.
- The perfect entry point for people who want basic yet wholesome cooking methods suitable for their daily activities.
- Each recipe provides weight loss support through dishes that help you manage your SmartPoints range without losing satisfaction and staying full.
- Building confidence becomes possible when you acquire knowledge and skills about better daily food decisions.
- Losing weight brings you physical wellness together with emotional well-being and a sensational feeling of being your best.
- Learning to harness the SmartPoints System means understanding its points system for healthy selection.
- The guide shows users easy ways to produce tasty low-point home-cooked meals.
- Discover steps that will maintain your motivation while also knowing how to reward yourself for your achievements.
- Making healthy eating a permanent joyful aspect of your life constitutes an effective life transformation for you.

Unlocking the Power of the WW SmartPoints System

Everyone agrees that eating healthy becomes a complex challenge. People get easily lost among different food diets and nutritional data that need tracking. The WW SmartPoints System serves as the main tool for users seeking balance. The SmartPoints System serves as a transformative instrument that helps people develop stress-free balanced healthier lives through nutrition.

What Are SmartPoints?

The SmartPoints system defines a measurement standard to calculate nutritional values found in eaten foods. SmartPoints move past traditional calorie counting because they evaluate food through a combination of saturated fat along with sugar and calorie values. Food products containing sugar along with saturated fat will accumulate more SmartPoints than protein-rich and fiber-rich foods. This system helps people choose better healthier options while eliminating feelings of dietary restriction.

Why SmartPoints Work

1. The Weight Watchers dietary program assigns SmartPoints to all foods including apples along with pizza and every tiny piece of nutrition gets measured according to its profile.
2. WW assigns you a personal SmartPoints budget which computes from your age information combined with your weight and height alongside your physical activity level. The planning system adjusts the approach specifically toward your requirements.
3. The WW app combined with a personal food journal helps you maintain daily dietary choices because you need to track all your food consumption.

The effectiveness stems from the fact that point allocation focuses on achieving equilibrium instead of placing limits on food choices. The program lets you consume your desired foods so you can develop better dietary decisions to abide by your spending limit. The WW SmartPoints system lets you choose between a donut with 10 Points or a Greek yogurt with fresh berries totaling 2 Points.

How SmartPoints Simplify Meal Planning

Every food under the SmartPoints system carries its point value so that you can immediately check how your dishes match your daily spending limits.

- **Flexibility:** Craving pizza? No problem. Reaching your daily SmartPoints goal is possible by combining high-point meals with smaller meals containing fewer points during the day.
- SmartPoints training promotes food quality evaluation over simple portion measurement.
- When planning dinner, you can illustrate the use of SmartPoints. Using the SmartPoints system, you can select grilled chicken with roasted vegetables as dinner which contains fewer points values while allowing you to enjoy a small dessert afterward. This open system accommodates your goals because it allows you to stick to them without experiencing feelings of diet restriction.

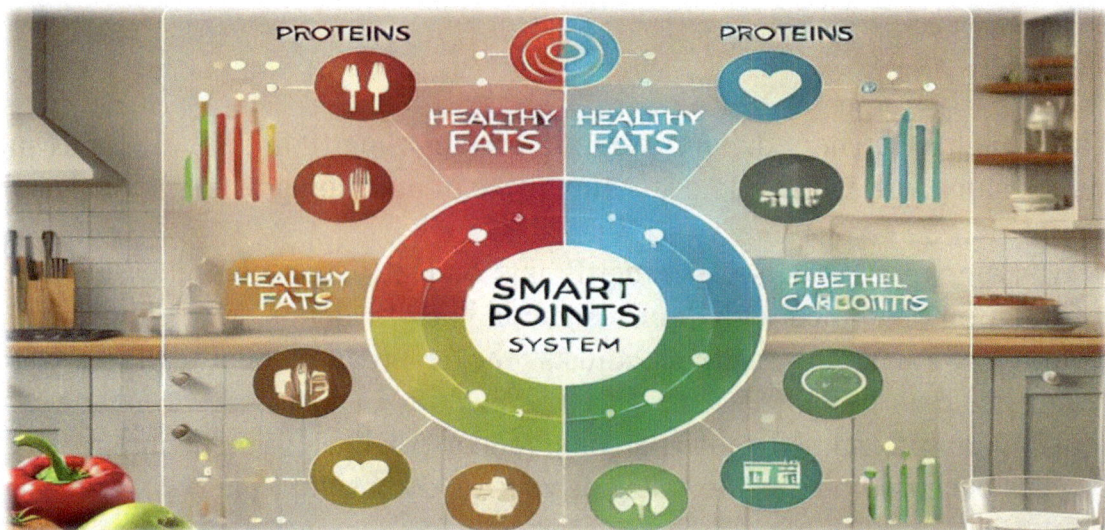

The Benefits of SmartPoints

- SmartPoints allows you to experience food pleasure without remorse through their method of teaching balanced habits between unhealthy and nutritious choices.
- Because the SmartPoints system focuses on long-term success, it provides sustainable weight loss outcomes that differ from fad diet results. Your goal here is not about temporary solutions but the development of permanent lifestyle practices.
- Your overall nutritional quality will grow better because you will concentrate on eating foods with lower sugar and saturated fat levels.
- Removing food-related stress is possible through SmartPoints by encouraging users to pause between bites while they focus on their food which leads to healthier eating patterns.

Real-Life Examples

- **Breakfast:** Opt for oatmeal with fresh fruit and a sprinkle of nuts instead of consuming sugary cereal (4 SmartPoints).
- **Lunch:** Swap a fast-food burger (15 SmartPoints) for a grilled chicken salad with a light dressing (6 SmartPoints).
- **Snacks:** The swap from chips to air-popped popcorn changes the points value from 7 SmartPoints down to 2 SmartPoints.

Through the WW SmartPoints System, you can achieve weight loss together with increased energy levels and self-assurance and ultimately better life healthfulness. This straightforward tool helps people eat healthily by creating a system that is both practical and satisfying for all types of eaters. Every person fresh to WW and experienced members will benefit from SmartPoints which guide smart meal decisions at each eating opportunity.

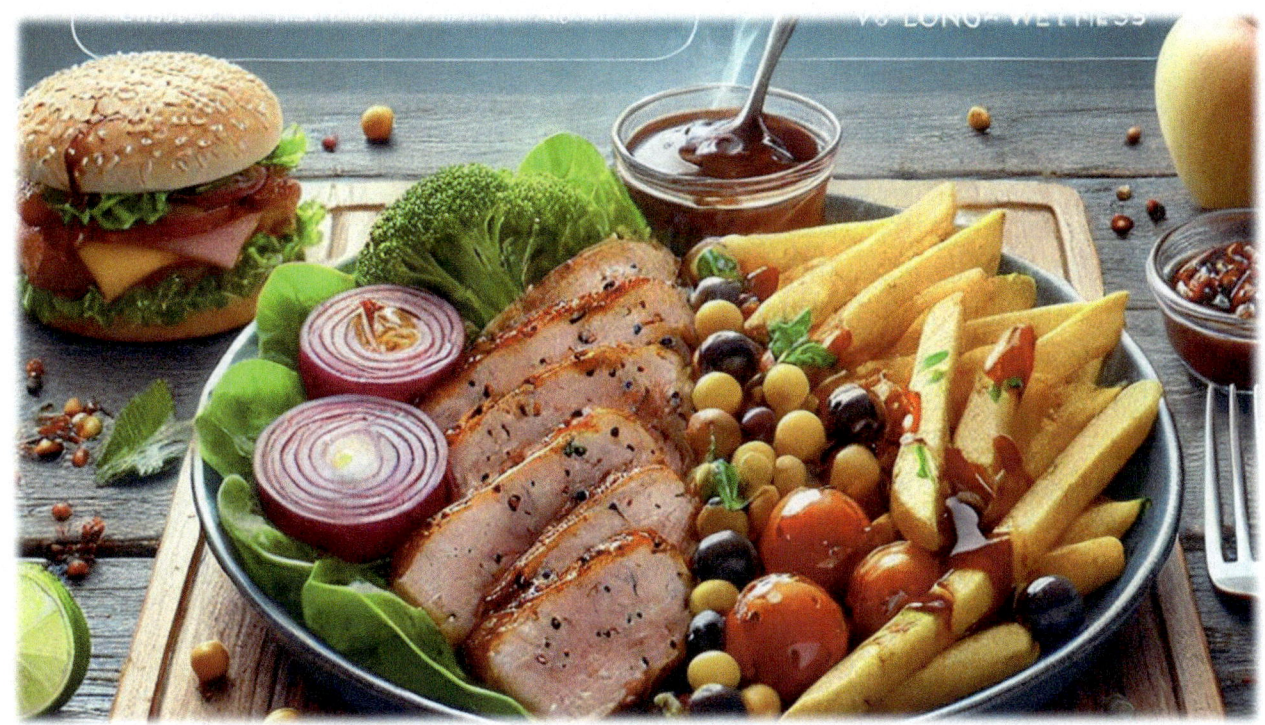

Why SmartPoints Are Key to a Balanced, Healthier Life

The SmartPoints system serves beyond its role as a tool through its ability to create a healthy life transition toward balance and wellness. Through both portion management and better food decisions this system directs you toward nutritionally beneficial items that back your wellness objectives.

A homemade stir-fry containing lean protein and veggies represents a better option than fast food because it contains only 6 SmartPoints compared to 15 SmartPoints of the fast-food meal.

The switching choice saves SmartPoints while removing the nutritional advantage and improving your feeding satisfaction duration. SmartPoints allows you to achieve weight management goals without suffering from food choice restrictions. The program allows you to eat your preferred foods when combined with wiser eating choices.

This approach to food improves how you relate to eating so that you can make conscious choices that benefit your ongoing health. SmartPoints serve as the essential tool through which you can reach a balanced healthier life whether you need to lose weight maintain your current weight or just want to eat better.

Setting Yourself Up for Success: A Guide to Starting Strong

A new start using the WW SmartPoints system can bring initial confusion but these guidelines will guide you into a confident beginning.

1. To start make objectives that are reachable through weekly weight loss of 1-2 pounds and preparing meals within your home.
2. Understand your food budget by learning the basics about SmartPoints assignment rules through the WW app. You should utilize the WW app to monitor your food consumption.
3. Using the SmartPoints system plan by developing weekly menus containing recipes that fit the system constraints. Preparation of ingredients beforehand will help save valuable time.
4. You should nurture your motivation through positive acknowledgments when you maintain your budget range or try preparing a nutritious dish.
5. Overcome Challenges:

    - Feeling hungry? Emphasize foods that have zero SmartPoints such as fruits and vegetables as a substitute for other food choices.
    - Craving sweets? Get a modest amount of pleasure food that matches your financial goals.
    - Eating out? Plan to examine the restaurant menu then pick meals that contain low SmartPoints values.

These measures will help you create a robust platform leading to your success. The road to progress demands patience because you need to provide yourself with self-kindness and understanding during the journey. You've got this!

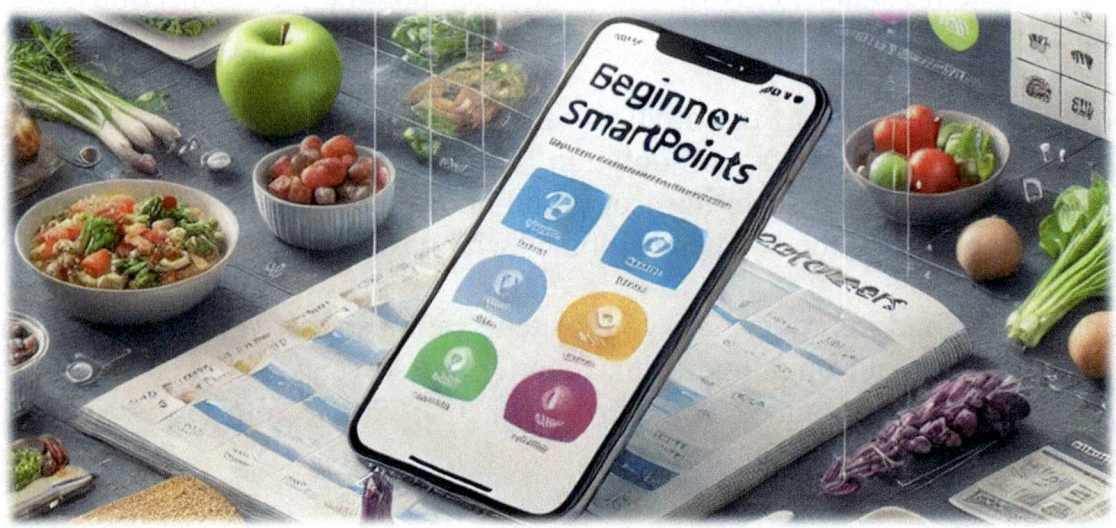

10 | *WEIGHT WATCHING* **SMARTPOINTS**

UNDERSTANDING SMARTPOINTS

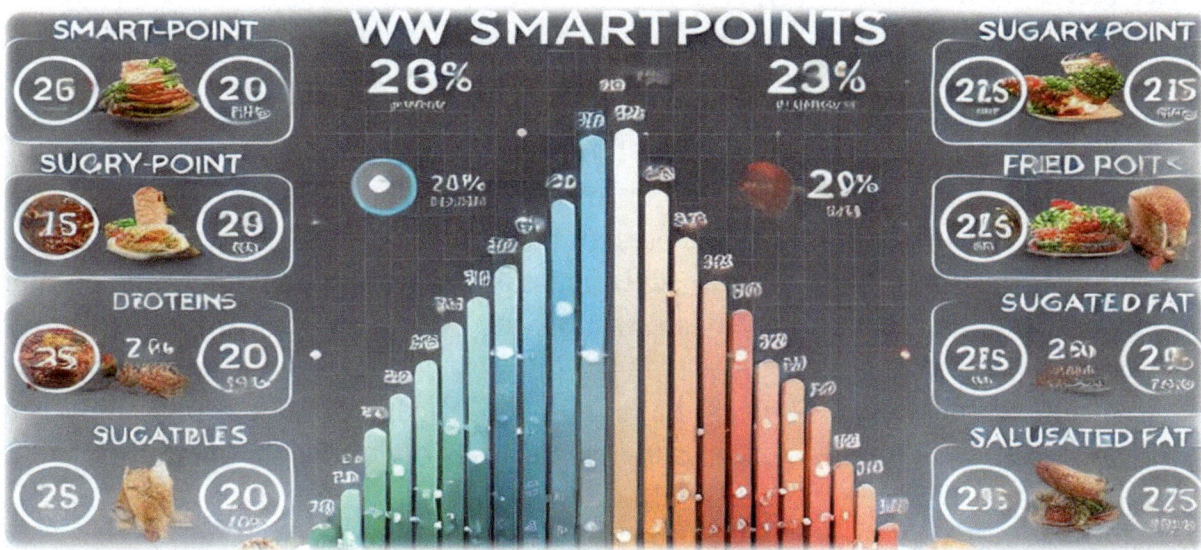

Demystifying SmartPoints: What You Need to Know

The WW SmartPoints System establishes a basic system for users to choose food items with better nutritional values. Traditional calorie tracking is different from SmartPoints because it bases points on food's nutritional value along with countable calories. The point system allocates values to foods through a system of calorie measurement together with saturated fat content and protein and sugar composition. Mountain-pointed foods contain sugar and saturated fats but low-pointed foods consist of protein along with fiber content.

For example:

- **High-point foods:** A slice of pepperoni pizza (12 SmartPoints) or a candy bar (10 SmartPoints).
- **Low-point foods:** Grilled chicken breast (1 SmartPoint) or a bowl of fresh fruit (0 SmartPoints).

You need to monitor SmartPoints either through the WW application or written meal logs in a journal. The weight management program determines your points through a combination of your age with weight height and activity level. Staying within your daily budget enables you to select multiple food options that support better decisions. The system reduces healthy food decisions to promote consideration of high-nutrient foods that also provide satisfaction. Using this system provides people with options to reach their wellness objectives while staying practical and flexible.

The Science Behind SmartPoints: How They're Calculated

The SmartPoints approach has scientific foundations that lead users toward making better food decisions. Here's how it works:

A formula determines SmartPoints by assessing four essential elements of a food:

1. **Calories:** The energy content of the food.
2. **Saturated Fats:** A higher number of SmartPoints exists for foods containing saturated fats since saturated fats present health risks.
3. **Sugar:** The SmartPoints system uses increased point values for foods containing sugar additives because they wish to motivate consumers toward controlling their sugar intake.
4. **Protein:** Professional choices have reduced SmartPoints because they supply protein which maintains satisfaction and supports body muscle operation.

For example:

- The combination of saturated fat and sugar content in donuts contributes to them earning a total of 10 SmartPoints worth.
- The SmartPoints value of a grilled salmon fillet amounts to 2 because this fish has both low sugar content and saturated fat levels and high protein content.

Through this approach, you have to select foods that offer fewer calories while providing more nutritional benefits. The knowledge about SmartPoints calculation enables you to make decisions that benefit your health and wellness needs.

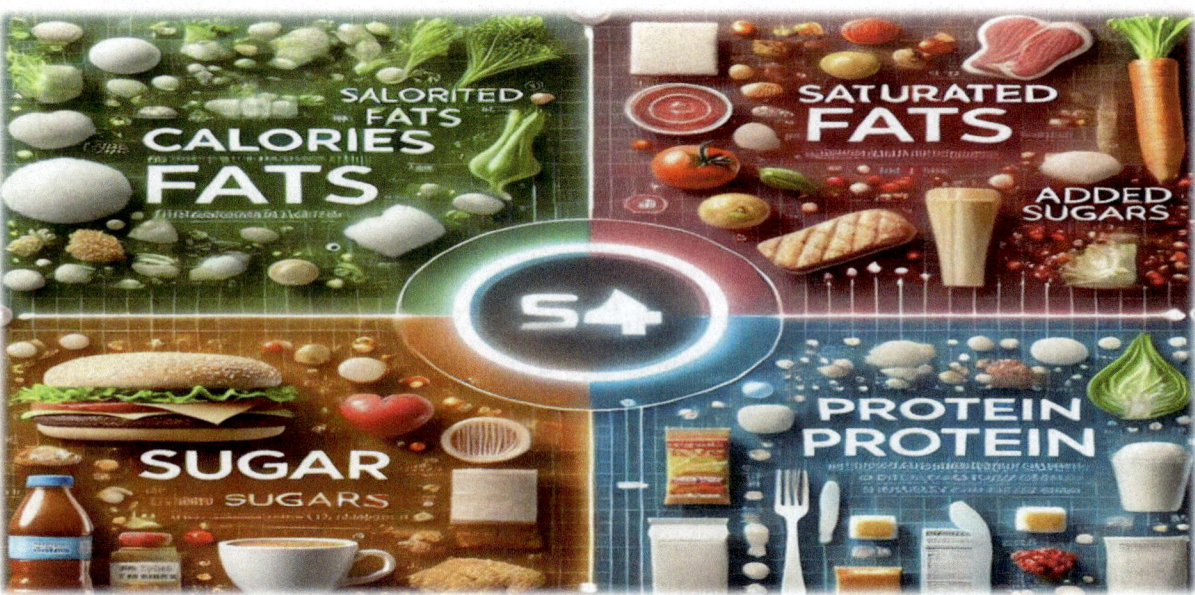

Using SmartPoints to Achieve Long-Term Wellness

The SmartPoints System helps people achieve weight loss alongside teaching habits which become essential for long-term health. A sustainable life plan becomes possible when you focus on being consistent with your eating habits while also practicing mindfulness and balance.

Here's how:

- Every day track your SmartPoints to maintain a clear understanding of your food decisions and achievement progress.
- Use SmartPoints as a tool to practice mindful eating which lets you select nutritious options that provide lasting satisfaction.
- Using SmartPoints in combination with exercise activities will create better energy levels and overall wellness.

When you experience sweet cravings, you can satisfy the desire with a small portion of dark chocolate because it equals three SmartPoints, but a candy bar would equal ten SmartPoints. Your numerous little changes across time transform into remarkable achievements in the pursuit of your goals.

Your individual life choices can be accommodated by the flexible nature of the SmartPoints system. Any social or mealtime situation supports wellness choices as you can pick foods that match your wellness goals.

The adoption of the SmartPoints System gives you more than nutritional modifications because it creates a complete life transformation. Take your initial step now to build a healthier lifestyle that will bring happiness into your life.

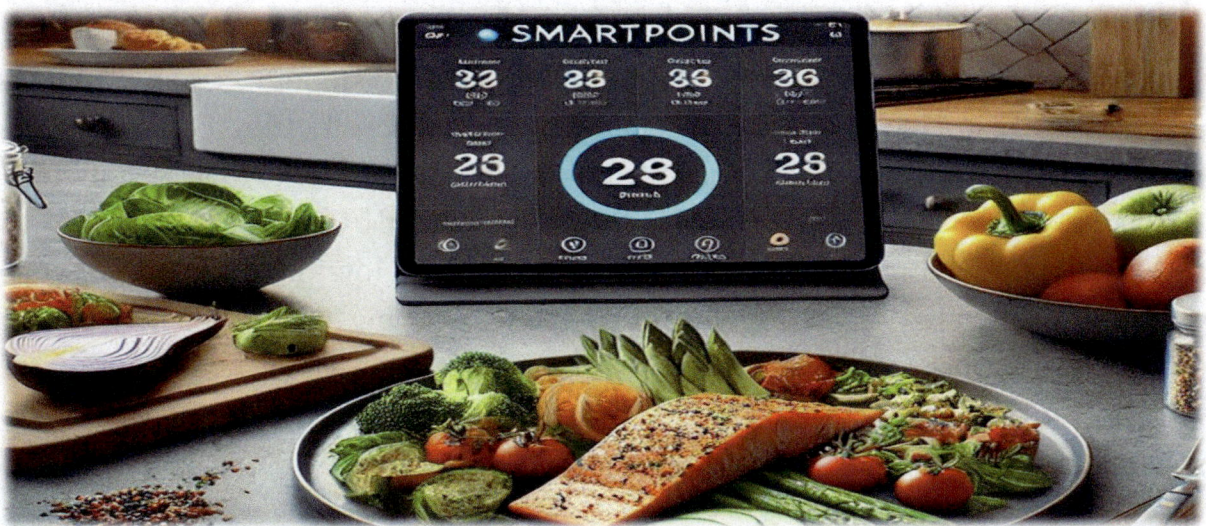

MASTERING YOUR SMARTPOINTS KITCHEN

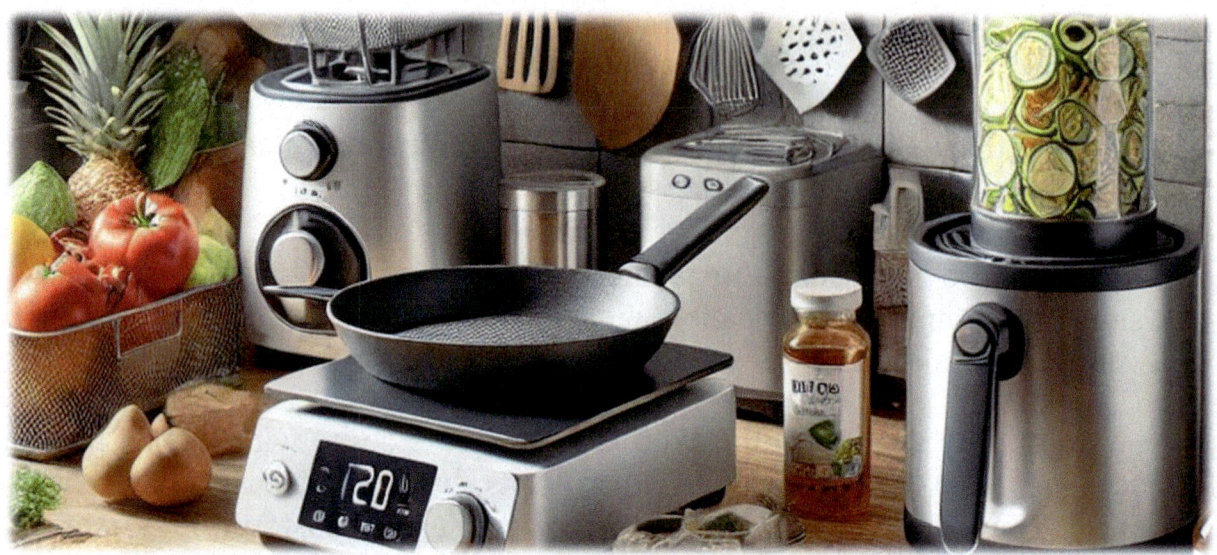

Essential Tools Every WW Kitchen Should Have

A few necessary kitchen devices will simplify your efforts at SmartPoints-friendly cooking:

- A non-stick skillet serves as an excellent kitchen tool because it lets you cook both oil-free and oil-light meals especially suitable for stir-fries or scrambled eggs.
- Using the food scale allows you to precisely measure portions to maintain your SmartPoints spending limit.
- The Blender serves as an excellent tool for preparing smoothies soups and sauces while using low-point ingredients including vegetables and fruits.
- The air fryer enables you to achieve crispy low-point snacks that include chicken tenders and roasted veggies because it offers healthier frying alternatives.
- Spiralizer: Turns veggies like zucchini into noodles, a low-point substitute for pasta.
- The measurement process requires accurate measuring tools both for baking and cooking purposes.
- You can cook large portions of low-point soups and stews with the help of a slow cooker which requires little work.

Stocking Your Pantry with SmartPoints-Friendly Staples

Your cooking success depends heavily on keeping important foods readily available in your pantry. Here's what to keep on hand:

- Brown rice together with quinoa and whole-wheat pasta serve as satisfying filling choices that maintain low SmartPoints value.
- The canned bean collection provides protein along with fiber which works well as an ingredient for salads soups and dips.
- Spice up your meals with low-point herbs and spices like garlic powder together with cumin and basil.
- Low-Sodium Broth: A base for soups and stews with minimal points.
- You should maintain a supply of popcorn combined with rice cakes and fresh fruits which are hearty and low in points.
- The healthy choice for oils includes olive oil together with cooking spray when used in moderate amounts.

Meal Ideas:

- **Breakfast:** Oatmeal with fresh fruit and a sprinkle of nuts.
- **Lunch:** Quinoa salad with beans, veggies, and a light vinaigrette.
- **Dinner:** Stir-fry with brown rice, lean protein, and plenty of veggies.

Your basic food supplies will prepare you for immediately preparing nutritious dishes in any situation.

Smart Shopping: How to Make Healthier Choices

The WW SmartPoints System does not require grocery shopping to be difficult. Follow these steps:

- Before you enter the supermarket create a list of items from your weekly dinner plans to stop yourself from buying spontaneous products.
- The calculation of SmartPoints requires reading product labels to find information about added sugars together with saturated fats and portion control.
- The perimeter area of the grocery store remains the ideal section because it contains fresh produce lean proteins and dairy products that have lower point values.

- Whole Foods provides the best option since you should pick whole grains along with fresh fruits and unprocessed veggies instead of processed food.
- Basic necessities such as beans spices and broth should be bought because they have lower SmartPoints.

SmartPoints-Friendly Shopping List:

- Fresh veggies (spinach, bell peppers, zucchini)
- Lean proteins (chicken breast, turkey, tofu)
- Whole grains (quinoa, brown rice)
- Low-point snacks (popcorn, Greek yogurt)

The tips provide a path to stock your shopping cart with items that adhere to your SmartPoints objectives.

Smart Prep: Time-Saving Tips for Meal Planning and Cooking

Preparation of your meals becomes your secret weapon for following the SmartPoints program. Here's how to make it work:

- Large quantities of staples such as grilled chicken alongside roasted veggies and quinoa should be cooked in advance for week-long use.
- Single-serving containers help portion control during meals to stop you from eating beyond your recommended amount.
- The preparation stage includes advanced chopping of veggies together with protein marinating and grain cooking which leads to efficient meal assembly time.
- A weeklong food schedule should include high- and low-point food selections to stay within your monetary budget constraints.

Weekly Meal Plan Example:

Breakfast: Greek yogurt with berries (2 SmartPoints).

Lunch: Grilled chicken salad with light dressing (5 SmartPoints).

Dinner: Stir-fry with tofu and veggies over brown rice (6 SmartPoints).

Snacks: Fresh fruit, air-popped popcorn, or rice cakes.

BREAKFAST DELIGHTS

1. Spinach & Mushroom Scramble with Feta

Ingredients:

- 1 cup fresh spinach
- 1/2 cup sliced mushrooms
- 2 large eggs
- (or 4 egg whites for fewer points)
- 1/4 cup crumbled feta cheese
- 1 tsp olive oil
- Salt and pepper to taste

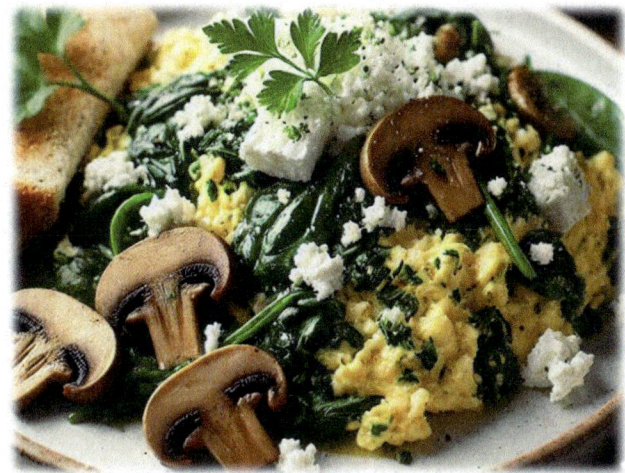

Cooking Time: 10 minutes

Instructions:

1. Heat olive oil in a non-stick skillet over medium heat.
2. Add mushrooms and sauté for 2-3 minutes until softened.
3. Add spinach and cook until wilted.
4. In a bowl, whisk eggs (or egg whites) with salt and pepper.
5. Pour eggs into the skillet and scramble until cooked through.
6. Sprinkle feta cheese on top and serve immediately.

2. Berry Almond Butter Smoothie

Ingredients:

- 1/2 cup unsweetened almond milk
- 1/2 cup mixed berries (strawberries, blueberries, raspberries)
- 1 tbsp almond butter
- 1/2 small banana (optional for sweetness)
- 1/2 cup ice

Cooking Time: 5 minutes

Instructions:

1. Add all ingredients to a blender.
2. Blend until smooth and creamy.
3. Pour into a glass and enjoy immediately.

3. Oatmeal with Fresh Fruit and Cinnamon

Ingredients:

- 1/2 cup rolled oats
- 1 cup water or unsweetened almond milk
- 1/2 cup fresh fruit (e.g., berries, sliced banana, or apple)
- 1/2 tsp cinnamon
- 1 tsp honey or sugar-free syrup (optional)

Cooking Time: 10 minutes

Instructions:

1. Cook oats with water or almond milk on the stovetop or microwave until thickened.
2. Top with fresh fruit, cinnamon, and a drizzle of honey or syrup if desired.

4. Avocado, Tomato & Egg Breakfast Bowl

Ingredients:

- 1/2 avocado, diced
- 1/2 cup cherry tomatoes, halved
- 1 boiled or poached egg
- Salt and pepper to taste
- 1 tsp lemon juice (optional)

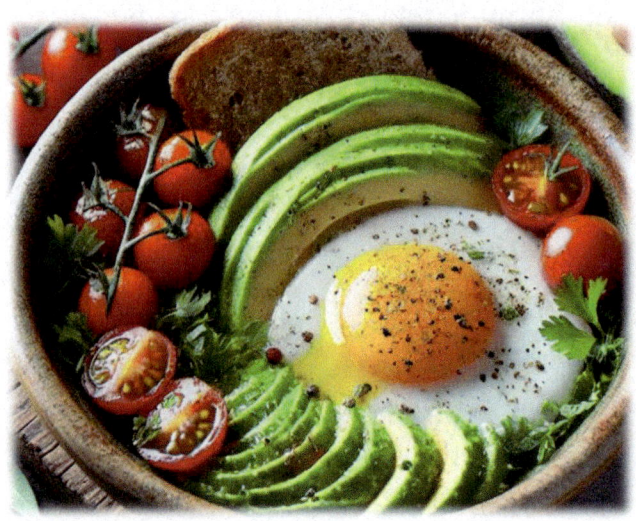

Cooking Time: 10 minutes

Instructions:

1. Boil or poach the egg to your desired doneness.
2. In a bowl, combine avocado and tomatoes.
3. Top with the egg, season with salt, pepper, and lemon juice.

5. Coconut Yogurt with Mango and Chia Seeds

Ingredients:

- 1/2 cup unsweetened coconut yogurt
- 1/4 cup diced mango
- 1 tsp chia seeds

Cooking Time: 2 minutes

Instructions:

1. Layer coconut yogurt, mango, and chia seeds in a bowl.
2. Serve immediately or refrigerate for a chilled treat.

6. Baked Egg Cups with Spinach & Cheese

Ingredients:

- 4 large eggs (or 8 egg whites)
- 1 cup fresh spinach, chopped
- 1/4 cup shredded low-fat cheese
- Salt and pepper to taste

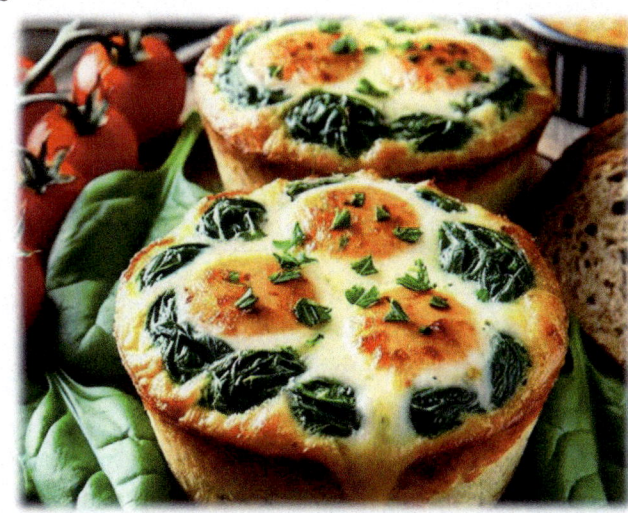

Cooking Time: 20 minutes

Instructions:

1. Preheat oven to 350°F (175°C).
2. Grease a muffin tin with cooking spray.
3. In a bowl, whisk eggs (or egg whites) with salt and pepper.
4. Add spinach and cheese to the egg mixture.

5. Pour into muffin cups and bake for 15-18 minutes until set.

7. Healthy Sweet Potato Breakfast Hash

Ingredients:

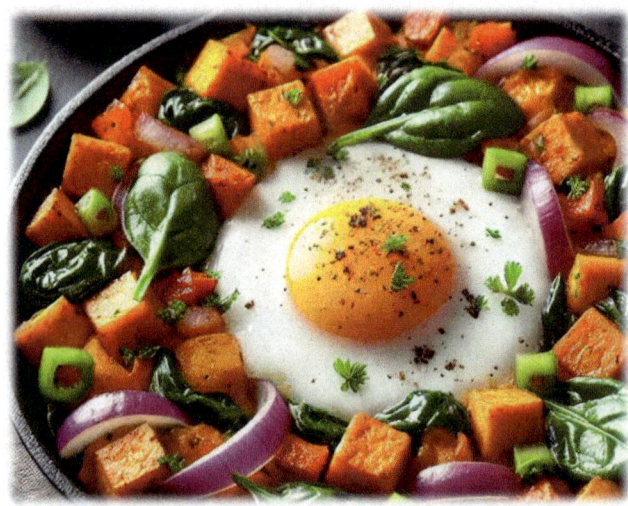

- 1 small sweet potato, diced
- 1/2 cup bell peppers, diced
- 1/4 cup onion, diced
- 1 tsp olive oil
- 1 egg (optional)
- Salt and pepper to taste

Cooking Time: 20 minutes

Instructions:

1. Heat olive oil in a skillet over medium heat.
2. Add sweet potato, peppers, and onion. Cook until tender, about 10-12 minutes.
3. Optional: Make a well in the hash, crack an egg into it, and cook until the egg is set.

8. Apple Cinnamon Quinoa Porridge

Ingredients:

- 1/2 cup cooked quinoa
- 1/2 cup unsweetened almond milk
- 1/2 apple, diced
- 1/2 tsp cinnamon
- 1 tsp honey or sugar-free syrup (optional)

Cooking Time: 10 minutes

Instructions:

1. Combine cooked quinoa and almond milk in a saucepan. Heat until warm.
2. Stir in diced apple and cinnamon.

3. Sweeten with honey or syrup if desired.

9. Protein-Packed Banana Pancakes

Ingredients:

- 1 ripe banana, mashed
- 2 eggs
- 1/4 cup oats
- 1/4 tsp cinnamon

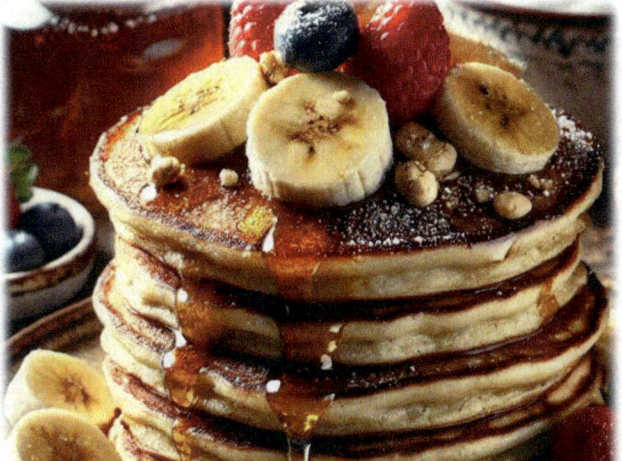

Cooking Time: 15 minutes

Instructions:

1. Mash banana in a bowl and whisk in eggs.
2. Stir in oats and cinnamon.
3. Heat a non-stick skillet over medium heat. Pour batter to form small pancakes.
4. Cook for 2-3 minutes per side until golden brown.

10. Scrambled Tofu and Veggie Breakfast Wrap

Ingredients:

- 1/2 cup firm tofu, crumbled
- 1/4 cup diced bell peppers
- 1/4 cup diced onion
- 1 whole wheat tortilla (low SmartPoints)
- 1 tsp olive oil
- Salt, pepper, and turmeric (optional for color)

Cooking Time: 15 minutes

Instructions:

1. Heat olive oil in a skillet. Sauté peppers and onion until soft.
2. Add crumbled tofu and season with salt, pepper, and turmeric. Cook for 5 minutes.
3. Spoon mixture onto a tortilla and wrap tightly.

21 | *WEIGHT WATCHING* SMARTPOINTS

11. Chia Seed & Fruit Parfait

Ingredients:

- 1/4 cup chia seeds
- 1 cup unsweetened almond milk
- 1/2 cup mixed berries
- 1 tsp honey (optional)

Cooking Time: Overnight (5 minutes prep)

Instructions:

1. Mix chia seeds and almond milk in a jar. Refrigerate overnight.
2. Layer chia pudding with berries in a glass. Drizzle with honey if desired.

12. Egg White & Veggie Breakfast Sandwich

Ingredients:

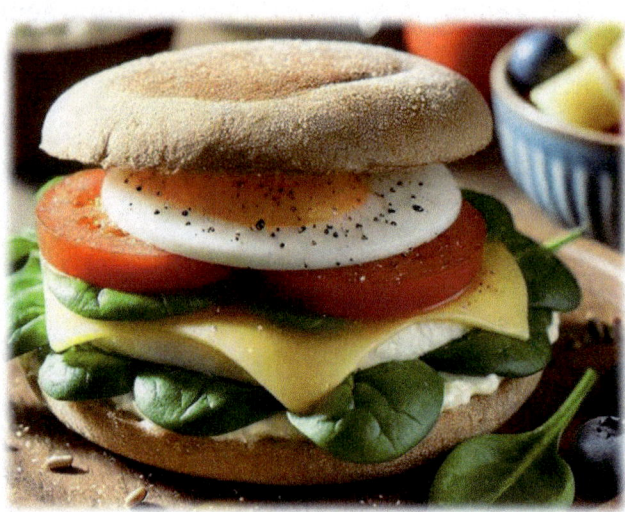

- 3 egg whites
- 1 whole wheat English muffin
- (low SmartPoints)
- 1/4 cup spinach
- 1 slice tomato
- 1 slice low-fat cheese (optional)

Cooking Time: 10 minutes

Instructions:

1. Cook egg whites in a non-stick skillet until set.
2. Toast the English muffin.
3. Layer egg whites, spinach, tomato, and cheese on the muffin.

13. Blueberry Almond Overnight Oats

Ingredients:

- 1/2 cup rolled oats
- 1/2 cup unsweetened almond milk

22 | *WEIGHT WATCHING* SMARTPOINTS

- 1/4 cup blueberries
- 1 tbsp almond butter
- 1 tsp chia seeds

Cooking Time: Overnight (5 minutes prep)

Instructions:

1. Combine oats, almond milk, and chia seeds in a jar.
2. Refrigerate overnight.
3. Top with blueberries and almond butter before serving.

14. Greek Yogurt & Granola Breakfast Cups

Ingredients:

- 1/2 cup non-fat Greek yogurt
- 1/4 cup low-SmartPoints granola
- 1/4 cup fresh fruit (e.g., berries or banana slices)

Cooking Time: 2 minutes

Instructions:

1. Layer Greek yogurt, granola, and fruit in a cup or bowl. Serve immediately.

15. Peach & Pecan Cottage Cheese Bowl

Ingredients:

- 1/2 cup low-fat cottage cheese
- 1/2 peach, sliced
- 1 tbsp chopped pecans
- 1 tsp honey (optional)

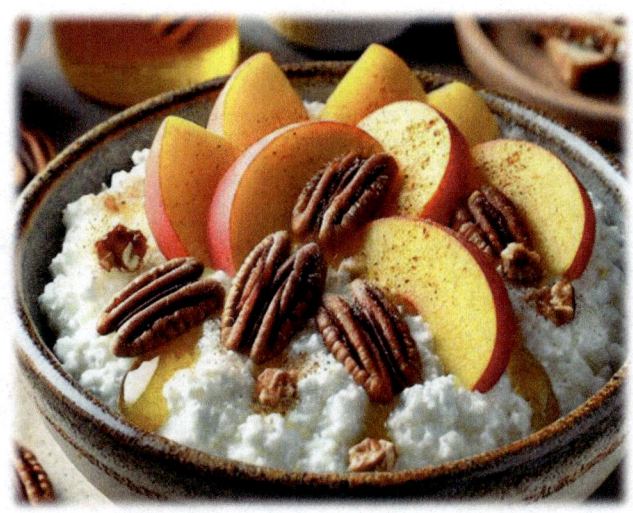

Cooking Time: 2 minutes

Instructions:

1. Place cottage cheese in a bowl.
2. Top with peach slices, pecans, and a drizzle of honey if desired.

23 | *WEIGHT WATCHING* **SMARTPOINTS**

SATISFYING SNACKS AND APPETIZERS

1. Spicy Baked Sweet Potato Wedges

Ingredients:

- 1 medium sweet potato, cut into wedges
- 1 tsp olive oil
- 1/2 tsp paprika
- 1/4 tsp cayenne pepper (adjust to taste)
- Salt and pepper to taste

Cooking Time: 25 minutes

Instructions:

1. Preheat oven to 400°F (200°C).
2. Toss sweet potato wedges with olive oil, paprika, cayenne, salt, and pepper.
3. Spread wedges on a baking sheet lined with parchment paper.
4. Bake for 20-25 minutes, flipping halfway through, until crispy.

2. Smoky Roasted Almonds with a Dash of Chili

Ingredients:

- 1 cup raw almonds
- 1/2 tsp smoked paprika
- 1/4 tsp chili powder
- 1/4 tsp garlic powder
- 1/4 tsp salt

Cooking Time: 15 minutes

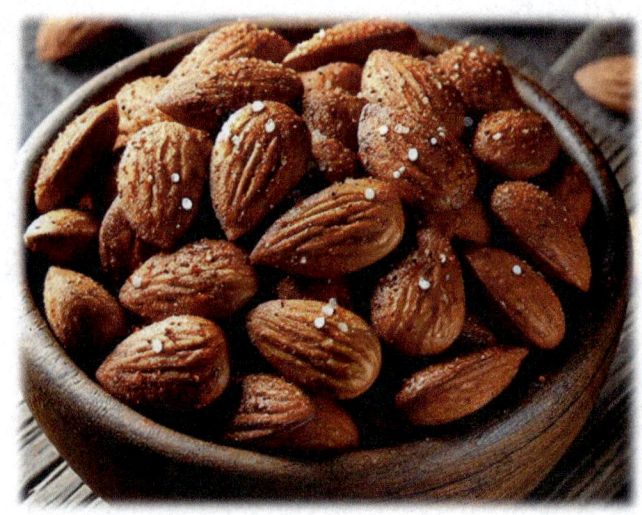

Instructions:

1. Preheat oven to 350°F (175°C).
2. Toss almonds with smoked paprika, chili powder, garlic powder, and salt.
3. Spread almonds on a baking sheet.
4. Roast for 10-12 minutes, stirring halfway through. Let cool before serving.

---

3. Crunchy Veggie Spring Rolls with Peanut Dipping Sauce

Ingredients:

- 4 rice paper wrappers
- 1/2 cup shredded carrots
- 1/2 cup cucumber, julienned
- 1/4 cup bell peppers, thinly sliced
- 1/4 cup fresh mint leaves
- 2 tbsp natural peanut butter
- 1 tbsp low-sodium soy sauce
- 1 tsp lime juice
- 1 tsp honey or sugar-free syrup

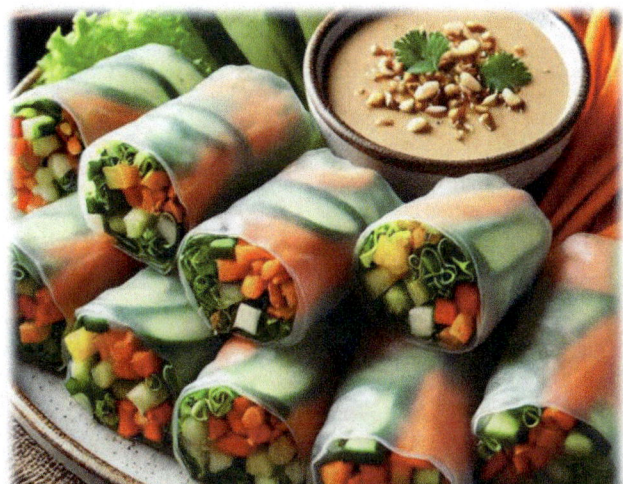

Cooking Time: 20 minutes

Instructions:

1. Dip rice paper wrappers in warm water to soften.
2. Layer carrots, cucumber, bell peppers, and mint in the center of each wrapper.
3. Fold sides and roll tightly.
4. For the sauce, whisk peanut butter, soy sauce, lime juice, and honey until smooth. Serve with spring rolls.

---

4. Crispy Baked Edamame with Sea Salt

Ingredients:

- 1 cup shelled edamame
- 1 tsp olive oil

25 | *WEIGHT WATCHING* SMARTPOINTS

- 1/4 tsp sea salt

Cooking Time: 20 minutes

Instructions:

1. Preheat oven to 400°F (200°C).
2. Toss edamame with olive oil and sea salt.
3. Spread on a baking sheet and bake for 15-20 minutes, stirring halfway through, until crispy.

---

5. Mini Caprese Salad Skewers with Balsamic Glaze

Ingredients:

- 8 cherry tomatoes
- 8 small mozzarella balls
- (bocconcini)
- 8 fresh basil leaves
- 1 tbsp balsamic glaze

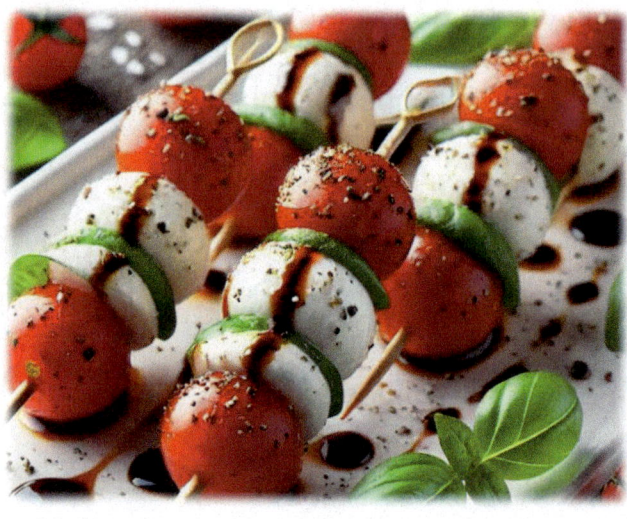

Cooking Time: 10 minutes

Instructions:

1. Thread a tomato, mozzarella ball, and basil leaf onto small skewers.
2. Drizzle with balsamic glaze before serving.

---

6. Zesty Guacamole with Baked Veggie Chips

Ingredients:

- 1 ripe avocado, mashed
- 1/4 cup diced tomato
- 1 tbsp lime juice
- 1 tbsp finely chopped red onion
- 1/4 tsp chili powder
- Salt to taste

- 1 cup sliced zucchini, sweet potato, or carrots (for chips)

Cooking Time: 25 minutes

Instructions:

1. For guacamole, mix avocado, tomato, lime juice, red onion, chili powder, and salt.
2. For chips, slice veggies thinly, toss with 1 tsp olive oil, and bake at 400°F (200°C) for 15-20 minutes until crispy. Serve with guacamole.

---

7. Cauliflower Buffalo Bites with Blue Cheese Dip

Ingredients:

- 2 cups cauliflower florets
- 1/4 cup hot sauce
- 1 tsp olive oil
- 1/4 cup non-fat Greek yogurt
- 1 tbsp crumbled blue cheese (optional)

Cooking Time: 25 minutes

Instructions:

1. Preheat oven to 425°F (220°C).
2. Toss cauliflower with olive oil and hot sauce. Spread on a baking sheet.
3. Bake for 20-25 minutes, flipping halfway through.
4. Mix Greek yogurt and blue cheese for dipping.

---

8. Stuffed Mushrooms with Spinach and Parmesan

Ingredients:

- 8 large mushrooms, stems removed
- 1/2 cup cooked spinach, chopped
- 2 tbsp grated Parmesan cheese
- 1/4 tsp garlic powder
- Salt and pepper to taste

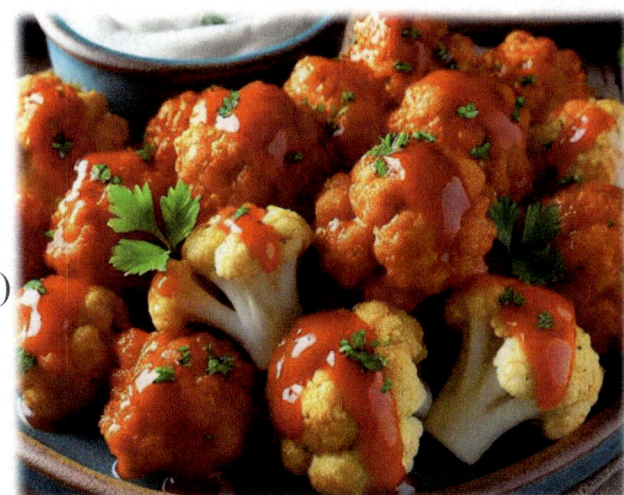

Cooking Time: 20 minutes

Instructions:

1. Preheat oven to 375°F (190°C).
2. Mix spinach, Parmesan, garlic powder, salt, and pepper.
3. Stuff mixture into mushroom caps.
4. Bake for 15-18 minutes until tender.

---

9. Chilled Shrimp Cocktail with Lemon-Dill Dip

Ingredients:

- 12 cooked shrimp, peeled and deveined
- 1/4 cup non-fat Greek yogurt
- 1 tbsp lemon juice
- 1/2 tsp fresh dill, chopped
- Salt and pepper to taste

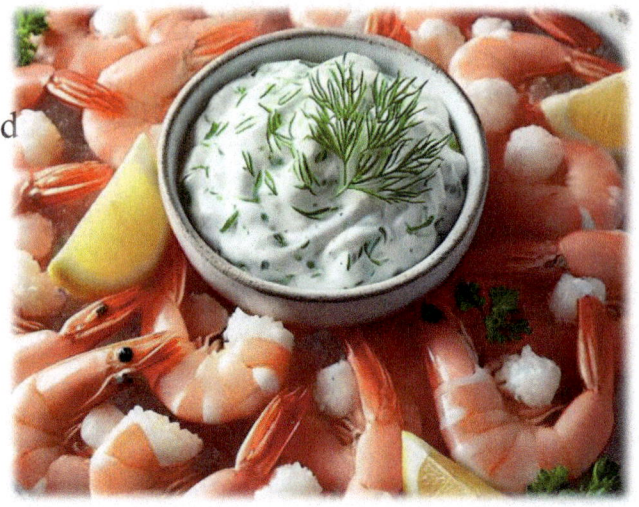

Cooking Time: 10 minutes

Instructions:

1. Combine Greek yogurt, lemon juice, dill, salt, and pepper for the dip.
2. Serve chilled shrimp with the dip.

---

10. Sweet & Savory Apple and Cheese Slices

Ingredients:

- 1 apple, sliced
- 1 oz low-fat cheddar cheese, sliced

Cooking Time: 5 minutes

Instructions:

1. Arrange apple and cheese slices on a plate.

2. Serve immediately.

11. Carrot and Cucumber Sticks with Hummus Dip

Ingredients:

- 1 cup carrot sticks
- 1 cup cucumber sticks
- 1/4 cup hummus

Cooking Time: 5 minutes

Instructions:

1. Serve carrot and cucumber sticks with hummus for dipping.

12. Crispy Parmesan Roasted Chickpeas

Ingredients:

- 1 cup canned chickpeas, drained and rinsed
- 1 tsp olive oil
- 2 tbsp grated Parmesan cheese
- 1/4 tsp garlic powder
- Salt to taste

Cooking Time: 30 minutes

Instructions:

1. Preheat oven to 400°F (200°C).
2. Toss chickpeas with olive oil, Parmesan, garlic powder, and salt.
3. Spread on a baking sheet and roast for 25-30 minutes, stirring halfway through, until crispy.

13. Greek Yogurt and Cucumber Dip with Pita Chips

Ingredients:

- 1/2 cup non-fat Greek yogurt
- 1/4 cup grated cucumber, drained

- 1/2 tsp garlic powder
- 1/2 tsp lemon juice
- Salt and pepper to taste
- 1 small whole wheat pita, cut into wedges

Cooking Time: 10 minutes

Instructions:

1. Mix Greek yogurt, cucumber, garlic powder, lemon juice, salt, and pepper.
2. Toast pita wedges in the oven or toaster until crispy. Serve with dip.

14. Avocado and Turkey Lettuce Wraps

Ingredients:

- 4 large lettuce leaves (e.g., romaine or butter lettuce)
- 4 slices lean turkey breast
- 1/4 avocado, sliced
- 1/4 cup shredded carrots
- 1 tbsp mustard or low-fat mayo (optional)

Cooking Time: 10 minutes

Instructions:

1. Lay lettuce leaves flat.
2. Layer turkey, avocado, and carrots on each leaf.
3. Drizzle with mustard or mayo if desired. Roll up and serve.

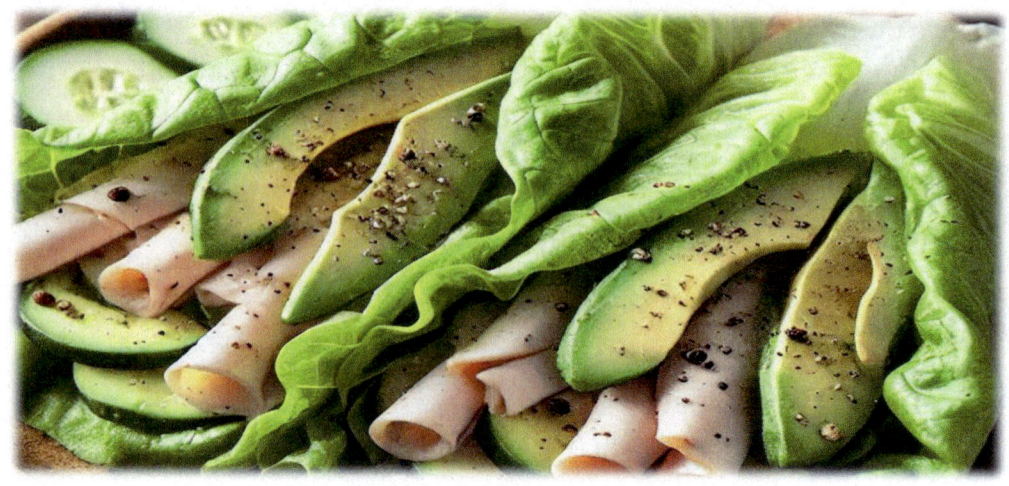

HEARTY SOUPS AND STEWS

1. Low-Calorie Chicken and Vegetable Soup

Ingredients:

- 1 lb boneless, skinless chicken breast, diced
- 4 cups low-sodium chicken broth
- 1 cup carrots, sliced
- 1 cup celery, sliced
- 1 cup zucchini, diced
- 1/2 cup onion, diced
- 1 clove garlic, minced
- 1 tsp olive oil
- Salt and pepper to taste
- 1 tsp thyme (optional)

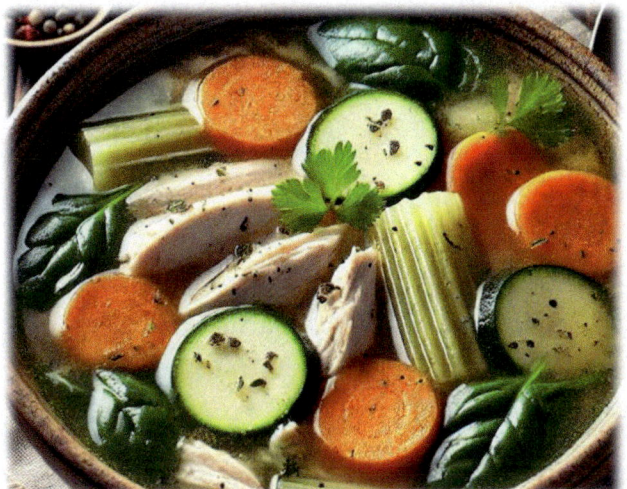

Cooking Time: 30 minutes

Instructions:

1. Heat olive oil in a large pot over medium heat. Sauté onion and garlic until softened.
2. Add chicken and cook until no longer pink.
3. Add broth, carrots, celery, zucchini, thyme, salt, and pepper.
4. Simmer for 20-25 minutes until vegetables are tender.

2. Spicy Lentil and Tomato Stew

Ingredients:

- 1 cup dried lentils, rinsed
- 4 cups low-sodium vegetable broth
- 1 can (14 oz) diced tomatoes
- 1/2 cup onion, diced
- 1/2 cup carrots, diced
- 1/2 cup celery, diced

WEIGHT WATCHING SMARTPOINTS

- 1 clove garlic, minced
- 1 tsp olive oil
- 1/2 tsp cumin
- 1/2 tsp chili powder
- Salt and pepper to taste

Cooking Time: 40 minutes

Instructions:

1. Heat olive oil in a pot over medium heat. Sauté onion, garlic, carrots, and celery until softened.
2. Add lentils, broth, tomatoes, cumin, chili powder, salt, and pepper.
3. Bring to a boil, then reduce heat and simmer for 30-35 minutes until lentils are tender.

---

3. Smart Points Beef and Barley Stew

Ingredients:

- 1/2 lb lean beef stew meat, trimmed
- 4 cups low-sodium beef broth
- 1/2 cup pearl barley
- 1 cup carrots, diced
- 1 cup celery, diced
- 1/2 cup onion, diced
- 1 clove garlic, minced
- 1 tsp olive oil
- 1 tsp thyme
- Salt and pepper to taste

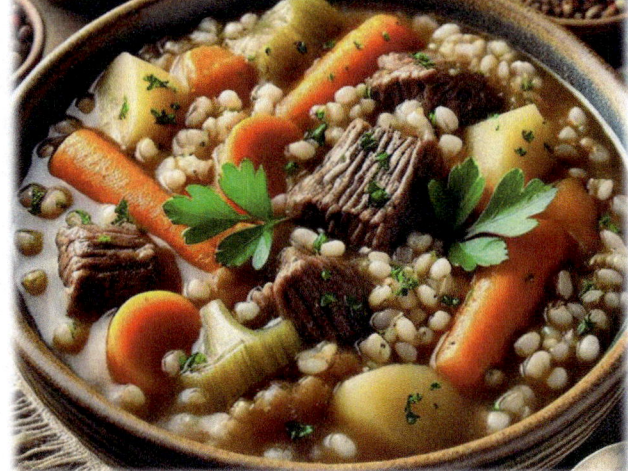

Cooking Time: 1 hour

Instructions:

1. Heat olive oil in a pot over medium heat. Brown beef on all sides.
2. Add onion and garlic, sauté until softened.
3. Add broth, barley, carrots, celery, thyme, salt, and pepper.
4. Simmer for 50-60 minutes until beef and barley are tender.

4. Creamy Cauliflower and Leek Soup

Ingredients:

- 1 head cauliflower, chopped
- 2 leeks, sliced (white and light green parts only)
- 4 cups low-sodium vegetable broth
- 1/2 cup unsweetened almond milk
- 1 tsp olive oil
- Salt and pepper to taste

Cooking Time: 30 minutes

Instructions:

1. Heat olive oil in a pot over medium heat. Sauté leeks until softened.
2. Add cauliflower and broth. Bring to a boil, then simmer for 20 minutes until cauliflower is tender.
3. Use an immersion blender to puree until smooth. Stir in almond milk, salt, and pepper.

---

5. Hearty Sweet Potato and Chickpea Stew

Ingredients:

- 1 large sweet potato, peeled and diced
- 1 can (15 oz) chickpeas, drained and rinsed
- 4 cups low-sodium vegetable broth
- 1/2 cup onion, diced
- 1 clove garlic, minced
- 1 tsp olive oil
- 1/2 tsp cumin
- 1/2 tsp smoked paprika
- Salt and pepper to taste

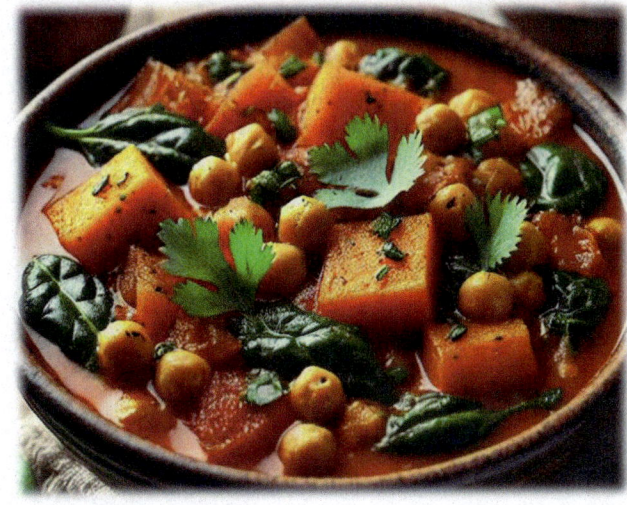

Cooking Time: 35 minutes

33 | *WEIGHT WATCHING* SMARTPOINTS

Instructions:

1. Heat olive oil in a pot over medium heat. Sauté onion and garlic until softened.
2. Add sweet potato, chickpeas, broth, cumin, smoked paprika, salt, and pepper.
3. Simmer for 25-30 minutes until sweet potatoes are tender.

---

6. Roasted Butternut Squash Soup with Sage

Ingredients:

- 1 small butternut squash, peeled and cubed
- 4 cups low-sodium vegetable broth
- 1/2 cup onion, diced
- 1 clove garlic, minced
- 1 tsp olive oil
- 1/2 tsp dried sage
- Salt and pepper to taste

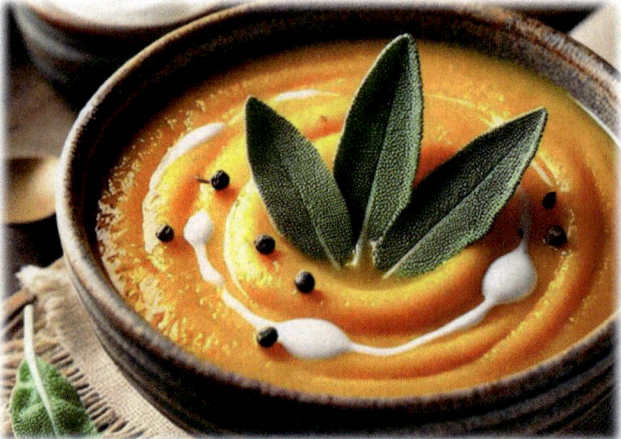

Cooking Time: 40 minutes

Instructions:

1. Preheat oven to 400°F (200°C). Toss butternut squash with olive oil and roast for 25 minutes.
2. In a pot, sauté onion and garlic until softened. Add roasted squash, broth, sage, salt, and pepper.
3. Simmer for 10 minutes, then blend until smooth.

---

7. Turkey and Kale White Bean Soup

Ingredients:

- 1/2 lb ground turkey
- 4 cups low-sodium chicken broth
- 1 can (15 oz) white beans, drained and rinsed
- 2 cups kale, chopped
- 1/2 cup onion, diced

- 1 clove garlic, minced
- 1 tsp olive oil
- Salt and pepper to taste

Cooking Time: 30 minutes

Instructions:

1. Heat olive oil in a pot over medium heat. Cook turkey until browned.
2. Add onion and garlic, sauté until softened.
3. Add broth, beans, kale, salt, and pepper. Simmer for 20 minutes.

---

8. Minestrone with Zucchini Noodles

Ingredients:

- 4 cups low-sodium vegetable broth
- 1 zucchini, spiralized into noodles
- 1/2 cup carrots, diced
- 1/2 cup celery, diced
- 1/2 cup onion, diced
- 1 clove garlic, minced
- 1 can (14 oz) diced tomatoes
- 1/2 cup cooked kidney beans
- 1 tsp olive oil
- Salt and pepper to taste

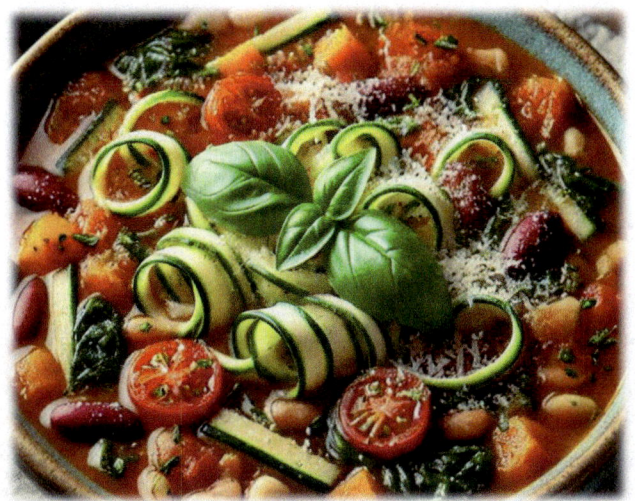

Cooking Time: 30 minutes

Instructions:

1. Heat olive oil in a pot over medium heat. Sauté onion, garlic, carrots, and celery until softened.
2. Add broth, tomatoes, beans, salt, and pepper. Simmer for 20 minutes.
3. Stir in zucchini noodles and cook for 2-3 minutes until tender.

---

35 | *WEIGHT WATCHING* **SMARTPOINTS**

9. Tomato Basil Soup with Grilled Cheese Croutons

Ingredients:

- 1 can (28 oz) crushed tomatoes
- 2 cups low-sodium vegetable broth
- 1/2 cup unsweetened almond milk
- 1/4 cup fresh basil, chopped
- 1 tsp olive oil
- Salt and pepper to taste
- 1 slice whole-grain bread, toasted and cut into cubes (optional)

Cooking Time: 25 minutes

Instructions:

1. Heat olive oil in a pot over medium heat. Add tomatoes, broth, salt, and pepper. Simmer for 15 minutes.
2. Stir in almond milk and basil. Blend until smooth if desired.
3. Serve with toasted bread cubes as croutons.

---

10. Chicken and Quinoa Stew with Lemon and Herbs

Ingredients:

- 1 lb boneless, skinless chicken breast, diced
- 4 cups low-sodium chicken broth
- 1/2 cup quinoa, rinsed
- 1/2 cup carrots, diced
- 1/2 cup celery, diced
- 1/2 cup onion, diced
- 1 clove garlic, minced
- 1 tsp olive oil
- 1 tbsp lemon juice
- 1 tsp thyme
- Salt and pepper to taste

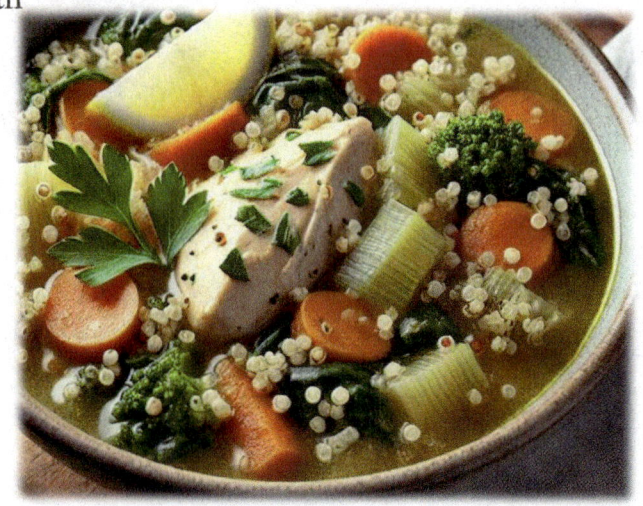

Cooking Time: 35 minutes

36 | *WEIGHT WATCHING* **SMARTPOINTS**

Instructions:

1. Heat olive oil in a pot over medium heat. Sauté onion, garlic, carrots, and celery until softened.
2. Add chicken and cook until no longer pink.
3. Add broth, quinoa, thyme, salt, and pepper. Simmer for 20-25 minutes.
4. Stir in lemon juice before serving.

---

11. Spicy Black Bean and Corn Soup

Ingredients:

- 1 can (15 oz) black beans, drained and rinsed
- 1 cup frozen corn
- 4 cups low-sodium vegetable broth
- 1/2 cup onion, diced
- 1 clove garlic, minced
- 1 tsp olive oil
- 1/2 tsp cumin
- 1/4 tsp chili powder
- Salt and pepper to taste

Cooking Time: 25 minutes

Instructions:

1. Heat olive oil in a pot over medium heat. Sauté onion and garlic until softened.
2. Add beans, corn, broth, cumin, chili powder, salt, and pepper.
3. Simmer for 20 minutes.

---

12. Roasted Carrot and Ginger Soup

Ingredients:

- 4 large carrots, peeled and chopped
- 4 cups low-sodium vegetable broth
- 1/2 cup onion, diced

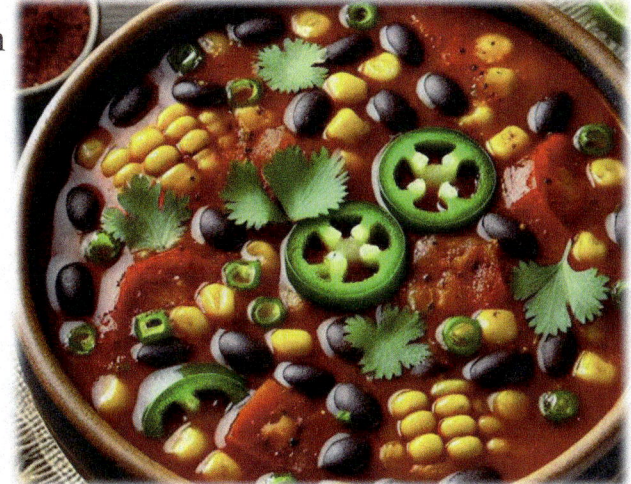

- 1 clove garlic, minced
- 1 tsp olive oil
- 1 tsp fresh ginger, grated
- Salt and pepper to taste

Cooking Time: 35 minutes

Instructions:

1. Preheat oven to 400°F (200°C). Toss carrots with olive oil and roast for 25 minutes.
2. In a pot, sauté onion, garlic, and ginger until softened.
3. Add roasted carrots and broth. Simmer for 10 minutes, then blend until smooth.

---

13. Vegetarian Chili with Avocado

Ingredients:

- 1 can (15 oz) kidney beans, drained and rinsed
- 1 can (15 oz) black beans, drained and rinsed
- 1 can (14 oz) diced tomatoes
- 1/2 cup onion, diced
- 1 clove garlic, minced
- 1 tsp olive oil
- 1/2 tsp cumin
- 1/2 tsp chili powder
- 1/4 cup avocado, diced (for topping)
- Salt and pepper to taste

Cooking Time: 30 minutes

Instructions:

1. Heat olive oil in a pot over medium heat. Sauté onion and garlic until softened.
2. Add beans, tomatoes, cumin, chili powder, salt, and pepper.
3. Simmer for 25 minutes. Top with avocado before serving.

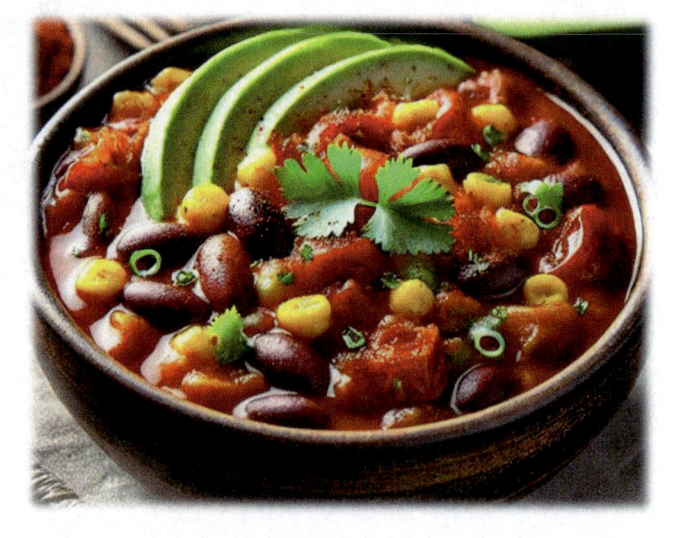

14. Healthy Beef and Cabbage Soup

Ingredients:

- 1/2 lb lean ground beef
- 4 cups low-sodium beef broth
- 2 cups cabbage, shredded
- 1/2 cup carrots, diced
- 1/2 cup onion, diced
- 1 clove garlic, minced
- 1 tsp olive oil
- Salt and pepper to taste

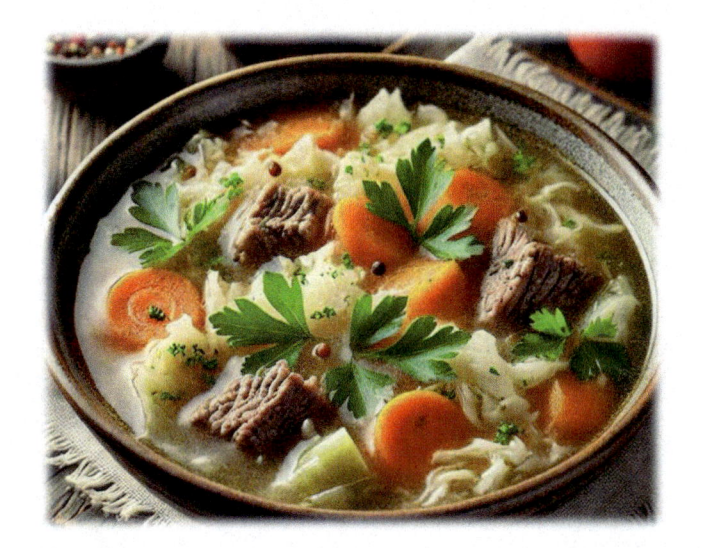

Cooking Time: 30 minutes

Instructions:

1. Heat olive oil in a pot over medium heat. Cook beef until browned.
2. Add onion, garlic, carrots, and cabbage. Sauté until softened.
3. Add broth, salt, and pepper. Simmer for 20 minutes.

15. Pumpkin and Coconut Milk Stew

Ingredients:

- 1 can (15 oz) pumpkin puree
- 1 cup light coconut milk
- 4 cups low-sodium vegetable broth
- 1/2 cup onion, diced
- 1 clove garlic, minced
- 1 tsp olive oil
- 1/2 tsp curry powder
- Salt and pepper to taste

Cooking Time: 25 minutes

Instructions:

1. Heat olive oil in a pot over medium heat. Sauté onion and garlic until softened.
2. Add pumpkin, coconut milk, broth, curry powder, salt, and pepper.
3. Simmer for 20 minutes, stirring occasionally.

WEIGHT WATCHING SMARTPOINTS

FLAVORFUL SALADS

1. Greek Salad with Grilled Chicken and Feta

Ingredients:

- 2 cups mixed greens
- 4 oz grilled chicken breast, sliced
- 1/4 cup cucumber, diced
- 1/4 cup cherry tomatoes, halved
- 1/4 cup red onion, thinly sliced
- 2 tbsp crumbled feta cheese
- 1 tsp olive oil
- 1 tbsp red wine vinegar
- Salt and pepper to taste

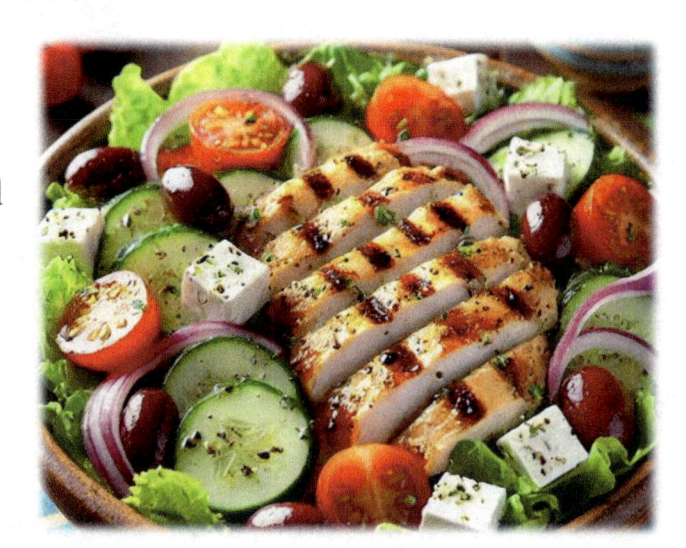

Cooking Time: 15 minutes

Instructions:

1. In a large bowl, combine mixed greens, cucumber, tomatoes, and red onion.
2. Top with grilled chicken and feta cheese.
3. Drizzle with olive oil and red wine vinegar. Season with salt and pepper.

---

2. Crispy Kale & Quinoa Salad with Lemon Tahini Dressing

Ingredients:

- 2 cups kale, chopped
- 1/2 cup cooked quinoa
- 1/4 cup shredded carrots
- 1 tbsp tahini
- 1 tbsp lemon juice
- 1 tsp olive oil
- 1/2 tsp garlic powder
- Salt and pepper to taste

Cooking Time: 10 minutes

Instructions:

1. Massage kale with olive oil until softened.
2. Add quinoa and carrots to the kale.
3. In a small bowl, whisk tahini, lemon juice, garlic powder, salt, and pepper. Drizzle over the salad.

---

3. Avocado and Black Bean Salad with Lime Vinaigrette

Ingredients:

- 1/2 avocado, diced
- 1/2 cup black beans, drained and rinsed
- 1/4 cup corn kernels
- 1/4 cup cherry tomatoes, halved
- 1 tbsp lime juice
- 1 tsp olive oil
- 1/4 tsp cumin
- Salt and pepper to taste

Cooking Time: 10 minutes

Instructions:

1. Combine avocado, black beans, corn, and tomatoes in a bowl.
2. Whisk lime juice, olive oil, cumin, salt, and pepper. Drizzle over the salad.

---

4. Zesty Cucumber & Tomato Salad with Fresh Herbs

Ingredients:

- 1 cucumber, sliced
- 1 cup cherry tomatoes, halved
- 1/4 cup red onion, thinly sliced
- 1 tbsp fresh parsley, chopped
- 1 tbsp fresh dill, chopped

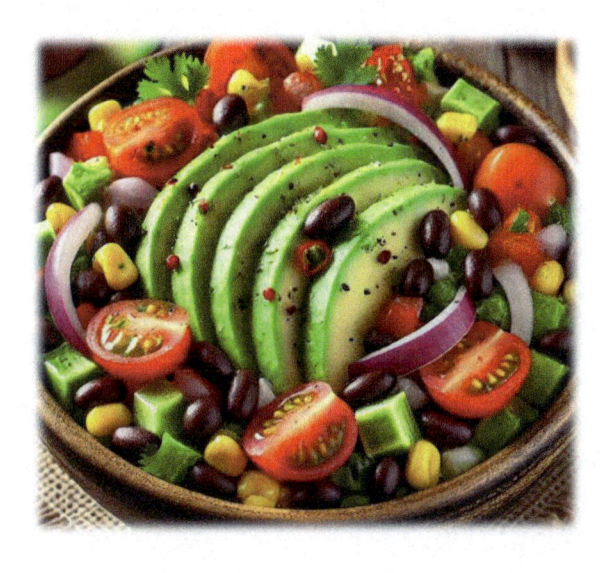

- 1 tbsp lemon juice
- 1 tsp olive oil
- Salt and pepper to taste

Cooking Time: 10 minutes

Instructions:

1. Combine cucumber, tomatoes, and red onion in a bowl.
2. Add parsley, dill, lemon juice, olive oil, salt, and pepper. Toss to combine.

---

5. Roasted Beet Salad with Arugula and Goat Cheese

Ingredients:

- 2 medium beets, roasted and sliced
- 2 cups arugula
- 1 oz goat cheese, crumbled
- 1 tbsp balsamic vinegar
- 1 tsp olive oil
- Salt and pepper to taste

Cooking Time: 40 minutes (including roasting)

Instructions:

1. Roast beets at 400°F (200°C) for 30 minutes. Let cool and slice.
2. Toss arugula with beets and goat cheese.
3. Drizzle with balsamic vinegar and olive oil. Season with salt and pepper.

---

6. Apple, Walnut, and Spinach Salad with Balsamic Glaze

Ingredients:

- 2 cups baby spinach
- 1/2 apple, thinly sliced
- 1 tbsp walnuts, chopped
- 1 tbsp balsamic glaze

- 1 tsp olive oil

Cooking Time: 10 minutes

Instructions:

1. Combine spinach, apple slices, and walnuts in a bowl.
2. Drizzle with balsamic glaze and olive oil.

---

7. Chopped Chickpea Salad with Cucumber and Red Onion

Ingredients:

- 1/2 cup chickpeas, drained and rinsed
- 1/2 cucumber, diced
- 1/4 cup red onion, diced
- 1 tbsp lemon juice
- 1 tsp olive oil
- 1/4 tsp paprika
- Salt and pepper to taste

Cooking Time: 10 minutes

Instructions:

1. Combine chickpeas, cucumber, and red onion in a bowl.
2. Whisk lemon juice, olive oil, paprika, salt, and pepper. Drizzle over the salad.

---

8. Mango and Avocado Salad with Cilantro Lime Dressing

Ingredients:

- 1/2 mango, diced
- 1/2 avocado, diced
- 1/4 cup red bell pepper, diced
- 1 tbsp fresh cilantro, chopped
- 1 tbsp lime juice
- 1 tsp olive oil

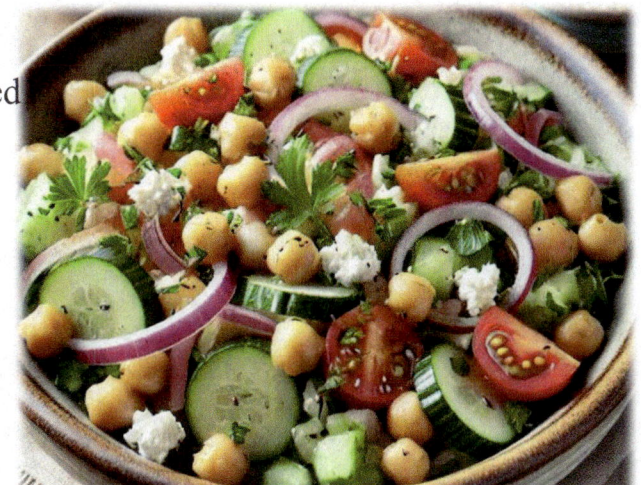

- Salt and pepper to taste

Cooking Time: 10 minutes

Instructions:

1. Combine mango, avocado, and bell pepper in a bowl.
2. Whisk cilantro, lime juice, olive oil, salt, and pepper. Drizzle over the salad.

---

9. Grilled Shrimp and Corn Salad with Cilantro-Lime Vinaigrette

Ingredients:

- 4 oz grilled shrimp
- 1/2 cup grilled corn kernels
- 2 cups mixed greens
- 1 tbsp lime juice
- 1 tsp olive oil
- 1 tbsp fresh cilantro, chopped
- Salt and pepper to taste

Cooking Time: 15 minutes

Instructions:

1. Combine mixed greens, shrimp, and corn in a bowl.
2. Whisk lime juice, olive oil, cilantro, salt, and pepper. Drizzle over the salad.

---

10. Sweet Potato, Kale, and Chickpea Salad with Dijon Dressing

Ingredients:

- 1 small sweet potato, roasted and diced
- 2 cups kale, chopped
- 1/2 cup chickpeas, drained and rinsed
- 1 tbsp Dijon mustard
- 1 tbsp apple cider vinegar
- 1 tsp olive oil

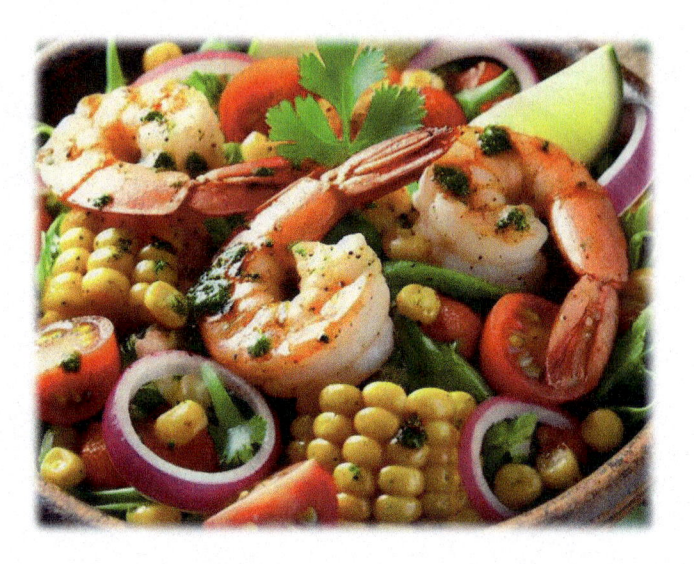

- Salt and pepper to taste

Cooking Time: 30 minutes

Instructions:

1. Roast sweet potato at 400°F (200°C) for 25 minutes. Let cool and dice.
2. Massage kale with olive oil until softened.
3. Combine kale, sweet potato, and chickpeas in a bowl.
4. Whisk Dijon mustard, vinegar, salt, and pepper. Drizzle over the salad.

---

11. Watermelon and Feta Salad with Fresh Mint

Ingredients:

- 1 cup watermelon, cubed
- 1 oz feta cheese, crumbled
- 1 tbsp fresh mint, chopped
- 1 tsp olive oil
- 1 tsp balsamic glaze

Cooking Time: 10 minutes

Instructions:

1. Combine watermelon, feta, and mint in a bowl.
2. Drizzle with olive oil and balsamic glaze.

---

12. Asian-Inspired Slaw with Sesame and Ginger Dressing

Ingredients:

- 2 cups shredded cabbage
- 1/2 cup shredded carrots
- 1 tbsp rice vinegar
- 1 tsp sesame oil
- 1/2 tsp fresh ginger, grated
- 1 tsp low-sodium soy sauce

45 | *WEIGHT WATCHING* SMARTPOINTS

- 1 tsp sesame seeds

Cooking Time: 10 minutes

Instructions:

1. Combine cabbage and carrots in a bowl.
2. Whisk rice vinegar, sesame oil, ginger, and soy sauce. Drizzle over the slaw.
3. Sprinkle with sesame seeds.

---

13. Cabbage and Carrot Slaw with Honey Mustard Dressing

Ingredients:

- 2 cups shredded cabbage
- 1/2 cup shredded carrots
- 1 tbsp Dijon mustard
- 1 tsp honey
- 1 tbsp apple cider vinegar
- 1 tsp olive oil
- Salt and pepper to taste

Cooking Time: 10 minutes

Instructions:

1. Combine cabbage and carrots in a bowl.
2. Whisk Dijon mustard, honey, vinegar, olive oil, salt, and pepper. Drizzle over the slaw.

---

14. Broccoli, Cauliflower, and Almond Salad with Yogurt Dressing

Ingredients:

- 1 cup broccoli florets
- 1 cup cauliflower florets
- 1 tbsp sliced almonds
- 2 tbsp non-fat Greek yogurt

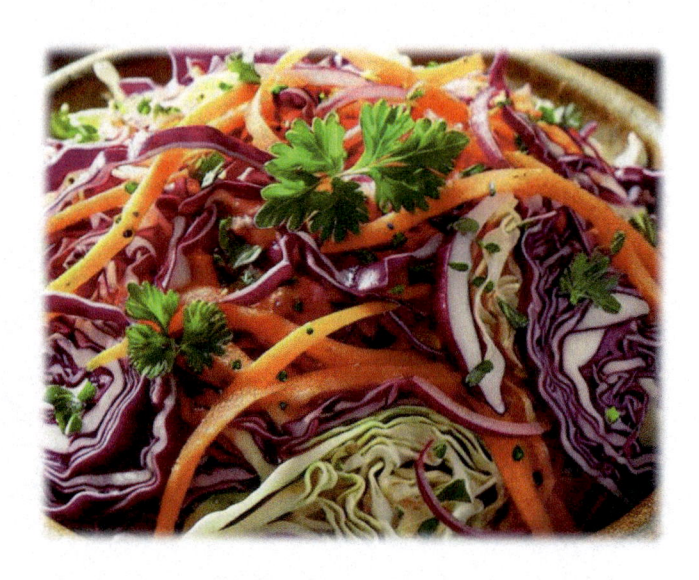

- 1 tsp lemon juice
- 1/2 tsp garlic powder
- Salt and pepper to taste

Cooking Time: 10 minutes

Instructions:

1. Combine broccoli, cauliflower, and almonds in a bowl.
2. Whisk yogurt, lemon juice, garlic powder, salt, and pepper. Drizzle over the salad.

15. Strawberry and Spinach Salad with Poppy Seed Dressing

Ingredients:

- 2 cups baby spinach
- 1/2 cup strawberries, sliced
- 1 tbsp slivered almonds
- 1 tbsp apple cider vinegar
- 1 tsp olive oil
- 1/2 tsp poppy seeds
- 1 tsp honey

Cooking Time: 10 minutes

Instructions:

1. Combine spinach, strawberries, and almonds in a bowl.
2. Whisk vinegar, olive oil, poppy seeds, and honey. Drizzle over the salad.

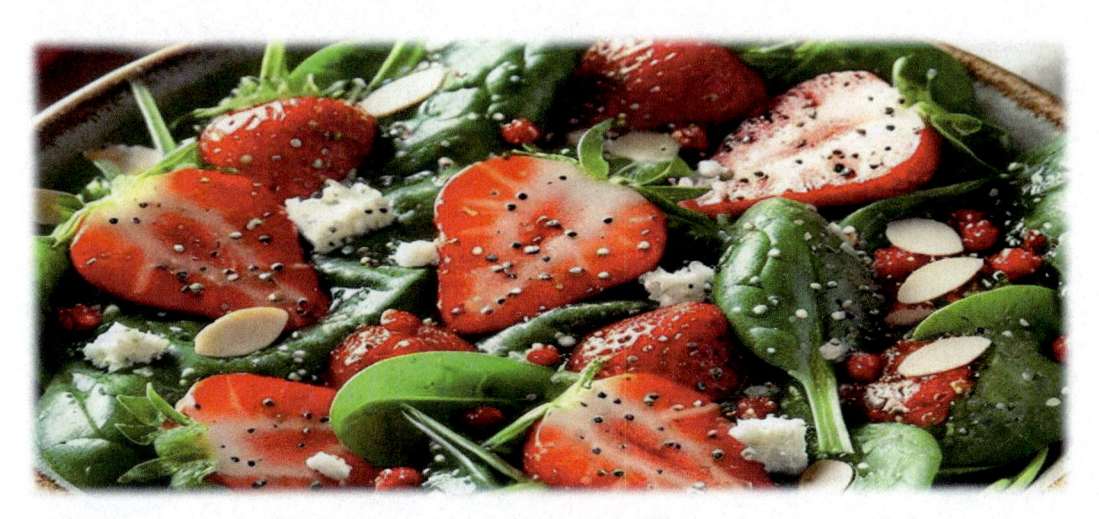

SEAFOOD

1. Grilled Lemon Herb Salmon

Ingredients:

- 2 salmon fillets (4 oz each)
- 1 tbsp lemon juice
- 1 tsp olive oil
- 1/2 tsp dried thyme
- 1/2 tsp dried oregano
- Salt and pepper to taste

Cooking Time: 15 minutes

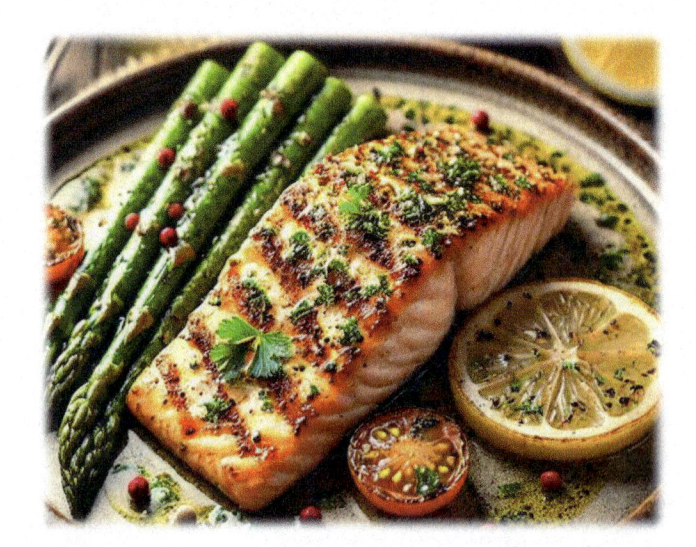

Instructions:

1. Preheat grill or grill pan to medium-high heat.
2. Brush salmon with olive oil and lemon juice. Sprinkle with thyme, oregano, salt, and pepper.
3. Grill for 4-5 minutes per side until cooked through.

---

2. Crispy Baked Fish Tacos with Avocado Slaw

Ingredients:

- 2 white fish fillets (e.g., cod or tilapia, 4 oz each)
- 1/2 cup panko breadcrumbs
- 1 tsp olive oil
- 1/2 avocado, mashed
- 1 cup shredded cabbage
- 1 tbsp lime juice
- 2 small whole wheat tortillas (low SmartPoints)
- Salt and pepper to taste

Cooking Time: 20 minutes

48 | WEIGHT WATCHING SMARTPOINTS

Instructions:

1. Preheat oven to 400°F (200°C).
2. Coat fish with panko breadcrumbs and place on a baking sheet. Drizzle with olive oil.
3. Bake for 12-15 minutes until crispy.
4. Mix mashed avocado, cabbage, and lime juice for the slaw.
5. Assemble tacos with fish and slaw.

3. Smart Shrimp Scampi with Zoodles

Ingredients:

- 8 oz shrimp, peeled and deveined
- 2 cups zucchini noodles (zoodles)
- 1 clove garlic, minced
- 1 tsp olive oil
- 1 tbsp lemon juice
- 1 tbsp fresh parsley, chopped
- Salt and pepper to taste

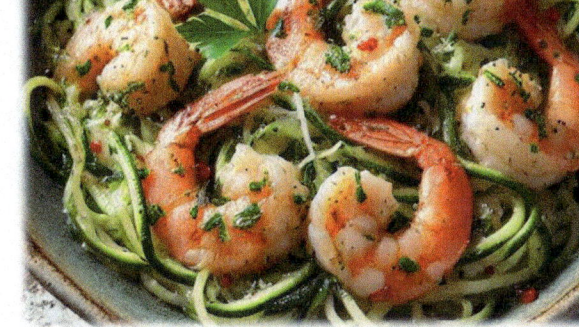

Cooking Time: 15 minutes

Instructions:

1. Heat olive oil in a skillet over medium heat. Sauté garlic until fragrant.
2. Add shrimp and cook until pink, about 3-4 minutes.
3. Add zoodles and lemon juice. Cook for 2-3 minutes until tender.
4. Sprinkle with parsley, salt, and pepper.

4. Spicy Sriracha Tuna Poke Bowl

Ingredients:

- 1/2 cup sushi-grade tuna, cubed
- 1/2 cup cooked brown rice
- 1/4 cup cucumber, diced
- 1/4 cup shredded carrots
- 1 tsp sriracha
- 1 tsp low-sodium soy sauce
- 1 tsp sesame seeds

49 | *WEIGHT WATCHING* **SMARTPOINTS**

Cooking Time: 10 minutes

Instructions:

1. In a bowl, combine tuna, sriracha, and soy sauce.
2. Layer brown rice, cucumber, and carrots in a bowl.
3. Top with tuna mixture and sprinkle with sesame seeds.

5. Garlic Butter Shrimp & Asparagus

Ingredients:

- 8 oz shrimp, peeled and deveined
- 1 cup asparagus, trimmed
- 1 clove garlic, minced
- 1 tsp olive oil
- 1 tsp light butter
- Salt and pepper to taste

Cooking Time: 15 minutes

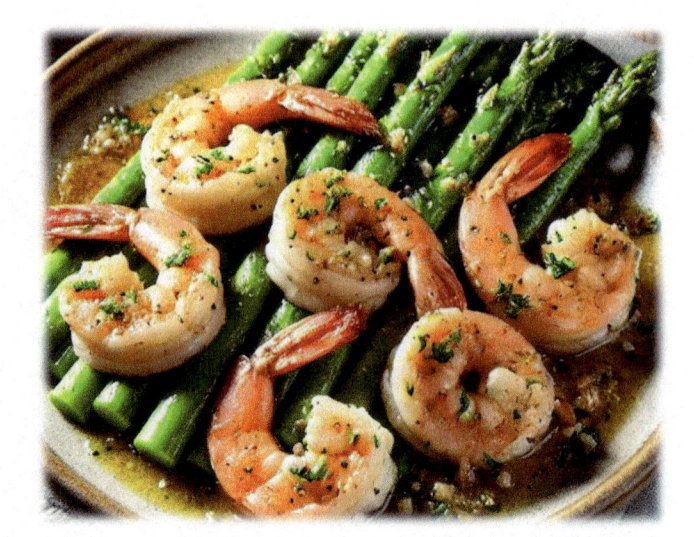

Instructions:

1. Heat olive oil and butter in a skillet over medium heat. Sauté garlic until fragrant.
2. Add shrimp and asparagus. Cook for 5-7 minutes until shrimp are pink and asparagus is tender.
3. Season with salt and pepper.

6. Miso Glazed Salmon with Steamed Vegetables

Ingredients:

- 2 salmon fillets (4 oz each)
- 1 tbsp miso paste
- 1 tsp honey
- 1 tsp rice vinegar
- 1 cup mixed vegetables (e.g., broccoli, carrots, snap peas)

Cooking Time: 20 minutes

Instructions:

1. Preheat oven to 400°F (200°C).
2. Mix miso paste, honey, and rice vinegar. Brush over salmon.
3. Bake salmon for 12-15 minutes.
4. Steam vegetables and serve with salmon.

---

7. Zesty Baked Cod with Roasted Tomatoes

Ingredients:

- 2 cod fillets (4 oz each)
- 1 cup cherry tomatoes, halved
- 1 tbsp lemon juice
- 1 tsp olive oil
- 1/2 tsp dried oregano
- Salt and pepper to taste

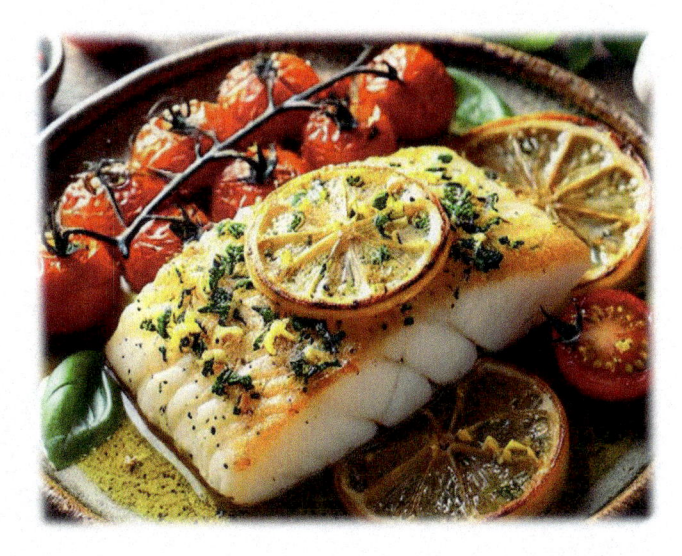

Cooking Time: 20 minutes

Instructions:

1. Preheat oven to 400°F (200°C).
2. Place cod and tomatoes on a baking sheet. Drizzle with olive oil and lemon juice.
3. Sprinkle with oregano, salt, and pepper.
4. Bake for 15-18 minutes until fish flakes easily.

---

8. Shrimp and Avocado Salad with Lime Dressing

Ingredients:

- 8 oz cooked shrimp
- 1/2 avocado, diced
- 2 cups mixed greens
- 1 tbsp lime juice
- 1 tsp olive oil
- Salt and pepper to taste

Cooking Time: 10 minutes

Instructions:

1. Combine shrimp, avocado, and mixed greens in a bowl.
2. Whisk lime juice, olive oil, salt, and pepper. Drizzle over the salad.

---

9. Mediterranean Tuna Salad with Feta and Olives

Ingredients:

- 1 can (5 oz) tuna in water, drained
- 1/4 cup cucumber, diced
- 1/4 cup cherry tomatoes, halved
- 1 tbsp crumbled feta cheese
- 1 tbsp Kalamata olives, sliced
- 1 tsp olive oil
- 1 tsp lemon juice

Cooking Time: 10 minutes

Instructions:

1. Combine tuna, cucumber, tomatoes, feta, and olives in a bowl.
2. Drizzle with olive oil and lemon juice.

---

10. Baked Tilapia with Cilantro Lime Rice

Ingredients:

- 2 tilapia fillets (4 oz each)
- 1/2 cup cooked brown rice
- 1 tbsp fresh cilantro, chopped
- 1 tbsp lime juice
- 1 tsp olive oil
- Salt and pepper to taste

Cooking Time: 20 minutes

52 | *WEIGHT WATCHING* **SMARTPOINTS**

Instructions:

1. Preheat oven to 400°F (200°C).
2. Place tilapia on a baking sheet. Drizzle with olive oil and lime juice. Season with salt and pepper.
3. Bake for 12-15 minutes.
4. Mix cooked rice with cilantro and serve with tilapia.

---

11. Crispy Fish Sticks with Tangy Tartar Sauce

Ingredients:

- 2 white fish fillets (e.g., cod or tilapia, 4 oz each)
- 1/2 cup panko breadcrumbs
- 1 egg, beaten
- 1 tbsp non-fat Greek yogurt
- 1 tsp Dijon mustard
- 1 tsp lemon juice
- Salt and pepper to taste

Cooking Time: 20 minutes

Instructions:

1. Preheat oven to 400°F (200°C).
2. Dip fish in beaten egg, then coat with panko breadcrumbs. Place on a baking sheet.
3. Bake for 15-18 minutes until crispy.
4. Mix yogurt, mustard, and lemon juice for the tartar sauce.

---

12. Seared Scallops with Lemon Garlic Sauce

Ingredients:

- 8 oz scallops
- 1 clove garlic, minced
- 1 tsp olive oil
- 1 tbsp lemon juice

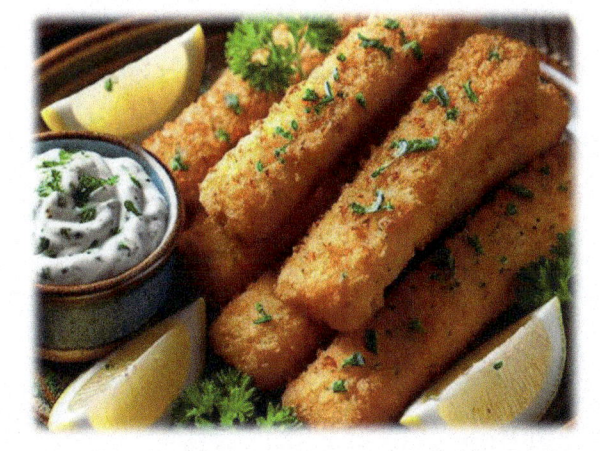

- 1 tbsp fresh parsley, chopped
- Salt and pepper to taste

Cooking Time: 10 minutes

Instructions:

1. Heat olive oil in a skillet over medium-high heat.
2. Season scallops with salt and pepper. Sear for 2-3 minutes per side until golden.
3. Add garlic, lemon juice, and parsley. Cook for 1 minute.

---

13. Coconut Crusted Shrimp with Sweet Chili Dip

Ingredients:

- 8 oz shrimp, peeled and deveined
- 1/4 cup shredded coconut
- 1/4 cup panko breadcrumbs
- 1 egg, beaten
- 1 tbsp sweet chili sauce
- 1 tsp lime juice

Cooking Time: 15 minutes

Instructions:

1. Preheat oven to 400°F (200°C).
2. Dip shrimp in beaten egg, then coat with coconut and panko. Place on a baking sheet.
3. Bake for 10-12 minutes until crispy.
4. Mix sweet chili sauce and lime juice for dipping.

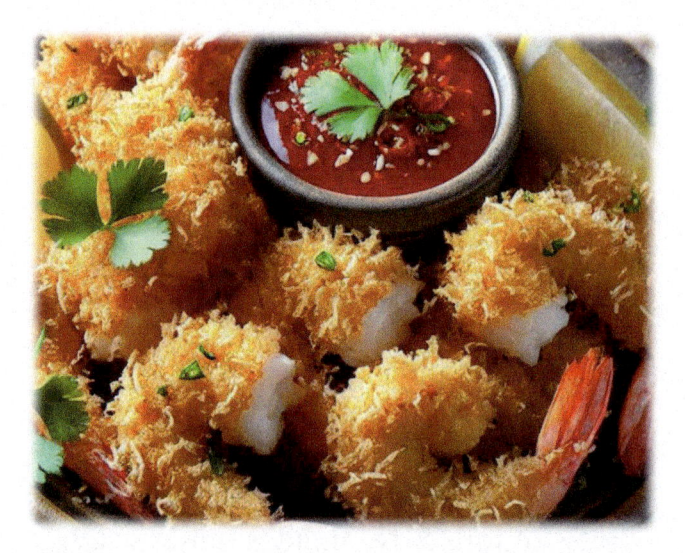

14. Salmon Patties with Dill Yogurt Sauce

Ingredients:

- 1 can (5 oz) salmon, drained
- 1/4 cup breadcrumbs
- 1 egg, beaten
- 1 tbsp fresh dill, chopped
- 2 tbsp non-fat Greek yogurt
- 1 tsp lemon juice
- Salt and pepper to taste

Cooking Time: 20 minutes

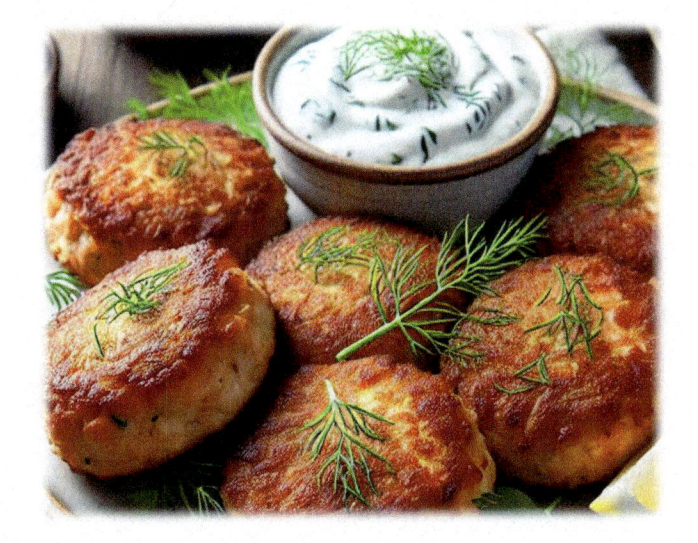

Instructions:

1. Mix salmon, breadcrumbs, egg, dill, salt, and pepper. Form into patties.
2. Cook in a non-stick skillet over medium heat for 4-5 minutes per side.
3. Mix yogurt and lemon juice for the sauce.

15. Seafood Paella with Brown Rice

Ingredients:

- 1/2 cup cooked brown rice
- 4 oz mixed seafood (e.g., shrimp, mussels, calamari)
- 1/4 cup diced tomatoes
- 1/4 cup bell peppers, diced
- 1 clove garlic, minced
- 1 tsp olive oil
- 1/2 tsp smoked paprika
- Salt and pepper to taste

Cooking Time: 25 minutes

Instructions:

1. Heat olive oil in a skillet over medium heat. Sauté garlic, tomatoes, and bell peppers.
2. Add seafood and cook until opaque.
3. Stir in cooked rice, smoked paprika, salt, and pepper. Cook for 5 minutes.

HEALTHY PLANT-BASED OPTIONS

1. Quinoa & Black Bean Stuffed Sweet Potatoes

Ingredients:

- 2 medium sweet potatoes
- 1/2 cup cooked quinoa
- 1/2 cup black beans, drained and rinsed
- 1/4 cup diced tomatoes
- 1/4 cup diced bell peppers
- 1 tbsp lime juice
- 1 tsp olive oil
- 1/4 tsp cumin
- Salt and pepper to taste

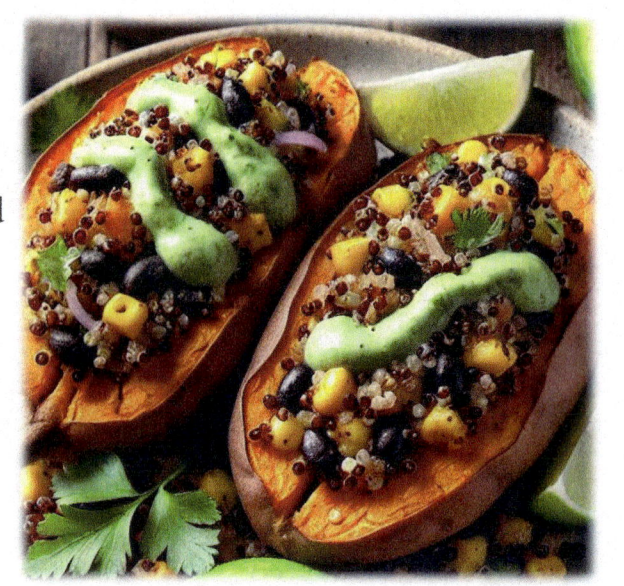

Cooking Time: 50 minutes

Instructions:

1. Preheat oven to 400°F (200°C). Pierce sweet potatoes and bake for 45 minutes until tender.
2. In a bowl, mix quinoa, black beans, tomatoes, bell peppers, lime juice, olive oil, cumin, salt, and pepper.
3. Slice sweet potatoes open and stuff with the quinoa mixture.

2. Lentil and Veggie Buddha Bowl

Ingredients:

- 1/2 cup cooked lentils
- 1/2 cup roasted vegetables (e.g., broccoli, carrots, zucchini)
- 1/2 cup cooked quinoa
- 1 tbsp tahini
- 1 tbsp lemon juice
- 1 tsp olive oil

- Salt and pepper to taste

Cooking Time: 30 minutes

Instructions:

1. Roast vegetables at 400°F (200°C) for 20 minutes.
2. Assemble lentils, roasted vegetables, and quinoa in a bowl.
3. Whisk tahini, lemon juice, olive oil, salt, and pepper. Drizzle over the bowl.

3. Chickpea Salad with Lemon Tahini Dressing

Ingredients:

- 1 cup chickpeas, drained and rinsed
- 1/2 cucumber, diced
- 1/4 cup cherry tomatoes, halved
- 1/4 cup red onion, diced
- 1 tbsp tahini
- 1 tbsp lemon juice
- 1 tsp olive oil
- Salt and pepper to taste

Cooking Time: 10 minutes

Instructions:

1. Combine chickpeas, cucumber, tomatoes, and red onion in a bowl.
2. Whisk tahini, lemon juice, olive oil, salt, and pepper. Drizzle over the salad.

4. Spaghetti Squash with Roasted Tomato and Pesto

Ingredients:

- 1 small spaghetti squash
- 1/2 cup cherry tomatoes, halved
- 1 tbsp basil pesto (low SmartPoints)
- 1 tsp olive oil
- Salt and pepper to taste

Cooking Time: 45 minutes

57 | *WEIGHT WATCHING* SMARTPOINTS

Instructions:

1. Preheat oven to 400°F (200°C). Cut spaghetti squash in half and remove seeds.
2. Place squash cut-side down on a baking sheet. Roast for 35-40 minutes.
3. Toss cherry tomatoes with olive oil, salt, and pepper. Roast for 15 minutes.
4. Scrape squash into strands and toss with pesto and roasted tomatoes.

5. Cauliflower and Chickpea Tacos with Avocado Salsa

Ingredients:

- 1 cup cauliflower florets
- 1/2 cup chickpeas, drained and rinsed
- 1/2 avocado, diced
- 1/4 cup diced tomatoes
- 1 tbsp lime juice
- 2 small whole wheat tortillas
- 1 tsp olive oil
- 1/2 tsp cumin
- Salt and pepper to taste

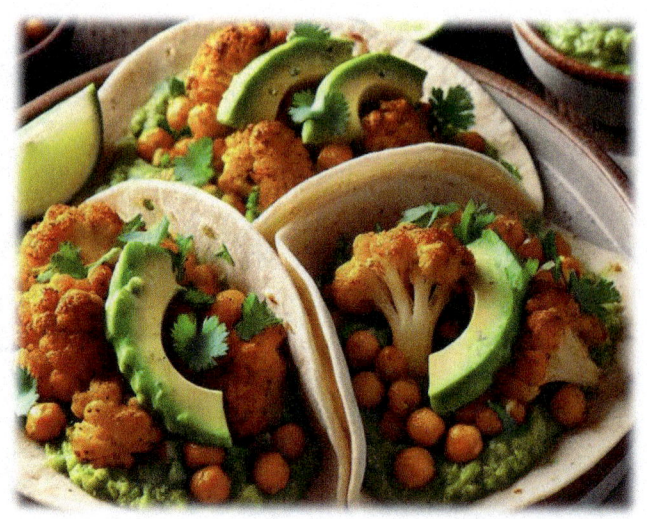

Cooking Time: 25 minutes

Instructions:

1. Preheat oven to 400°F (200°C). Toss cauliflower and chickpeas with olive oil, cumin, salt, and pepper. Roast for 20 minutes.
2. Mix avocado, tomatoes, and lime juice for the salsa.
3. Assemble tacos with roasted cauliflower, chickpeas, and avocado salsa.

6. Spicy Tempeh Stir-Fry with Veggies

Ingredients:

- 4 oz tempeh, cubed
- 1 cup mixed vegetables (e.g., bell peppers, broccoli, snap peas)
- 1 tbsp low-sodium soy sauce
- 1 tsp sriracha
- 1 tsp olive oil
- 1 clove garlic, minced

WEIGHT WATCHING **SMARTPOINTS**

Cooking Time: 20 minutes

Instructions:

1. Heat olive oil in a skillet over medium heat. Sauté garlic until fragrant.
2. Add tempeh and cook until golden, about 5 minutes.
3. Add vegetables, soy sauce, and sriracha. Stir-fry for 5-7 minutes until tender.

7. Vegan Cauliflower "Buffalo Wings"

Ingredients:

- 2 cups cauliflower florets
- 1/4 cup hot sauce
- 1 tsp olive oil
- 1/4 cup non-fat Greek yogurt (or vegan alternative)
- 1 tbsp fresh chives, chopped

Cooking Time: 25 minutes

Instructions:

1. Preheat oven to 425°F (220°C). Toss cauliflower with olive oil and hot sauce.
2. Spread on a baking sheet and bake for 20-25 minutes, flipping halfway through.
3. Serve with yogurt and chives for dipping.

8. Zucchini Noodles with Garlic, Basil & Cherry Tomatoes

Ingredients:

- 2 cups zucchini noodles (zoodles)
- 1/2 cup cherry tomatoes, halved
- 1 clove garlic, minced
- 1 tbsp fresh basil, chopped
- 1 tsp olive oil
- Salt and pepper to taste

Cooking Time: 10 minutes

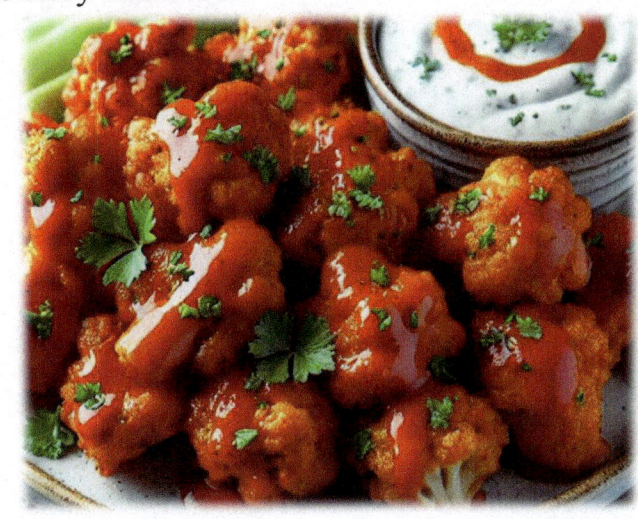

Instructions:

1. Heat olive oil in a skillet over medium heat. Sauté garlic until fragrant.
2. Add zoodles and cherry tomatoes. Cook for 3-4 minutes until tender.
3. Stir in basil, salt, and pepper.

9. Crispy Tofu Bites with Sriracha Lime Sauce

Ingredients:

- 1/2 block firm tofu, pressed and cubed
- 1 tbsp cornstarch
- 1 tsp olive oil
- 1 tbsp sriracha
- 1 tbsp lime juice
- 1 tsp honey or sugar-free syrup

Cooking Time: 20 minutes

Instructions:

1. Preheat oven to 400°F (200°C). Toss tofu with cornstarch and olive oil.
2. Bake for 15-20 minutes until crispy.
3. Whisk sriracha, lime juice, and honey for the sauce. Serve with tofu.

10. Roasted Vegetable and Quinoa Salad

Ingredients:

- 1 cup mixed vegetables (e.g., zucchini, bell peppers, carrots)
- 1/2 cup cooked quinoa
- 1 tbsp lemon juice
- 1 tsp olive oil
- Salt and pepper to taste

Cooking Time: 30 minutes

Instructions:

1. Preheat oven to 400°F (200°C). Toss vegetables with olive oil, salt, and pepper. Roast for 20 minutes.
2. Combine roasted vegetables with quinoa. Drizzle with lemon juice.

11. Sweet Potato and Black Bean Chili

Ingredients:

- 1 small sweet potato, peeled and diced
- 1/2 cup black beans, drained and rinsed
- 1/2 cup diced tomatoes
- 1/2 cup low-sodium vegetable broth
- 1/4 cup diced onion
- 1 clove garlic, minced
- 1 tsp olive oil
- 1/2 tsp chili powder
- 1/4 tsp cumin
- Salt and pepper to taste

Cooking Time: 30 minutes

Instructions:

1. Heat olive oil in a pot over medium heat. Sauté onion and garlic until softened.
2. Add sweet potato, black beans, tomatoes, broth, chili powder, cumin, salt, and pepper.
3. Simmer for 20-25 minutes until sweet potatoes are tender.

12. Vegan Lentil Shepherd's Pie

Ingredients:

- 1/2 cup cooked lentils
- 1/2 cup mixed vegetables (e.g., carrots, peas, corn)
- 1/2 cup mashed cauliflower (or mashed potatoes)
- 1/4 cup diced onion
- 1 clove garlic, minced
- 1 tsp olive oil
- 1/2 tsp thyme

- Salt and pepper to taste

Cooking Time: 40 minutes

Instructions:

1. Preheat oven to 375°F (190°C).
2. Heat olive oil in a skillet. Sauté onion and garlic until softened.
3. Add lentils, vegetables, thyme, salt, and pepper. Cook for 5 minutes.
4. Transfer to a baking dish and top with mashed cauliflower. Bake for 20 minutes.

13. Mango and Avocado Salad with Lime Dressing

Ingredients:

- 1/2 mango, diced
- 1/2 avocado, diced
- 2 cups mixed greens
- 1 tbsp lime juice
- 1 tsp olive oil
- Salt and pepper to taste

Cooking Time: 10 minutes

Instructions:

1. Combine mango, avocado, and mixed greens in a bowl.
2. Whisk lime juice, olive oil, salt, and pepper. Drizzle over the salad.

14. Coconut-Curry Chickpea Stew

Ingredients:

- 1 cup chickpeas, drained and rinsed
- 1/2 cup light coconut milk
- 1/2 cup diced tomatoes
- 1/4 cup diced onion
- 1 clove garlic, minced
- 1 tsp olive oil
- 1/2 tsp curry powder
- Salt and pepper to taste

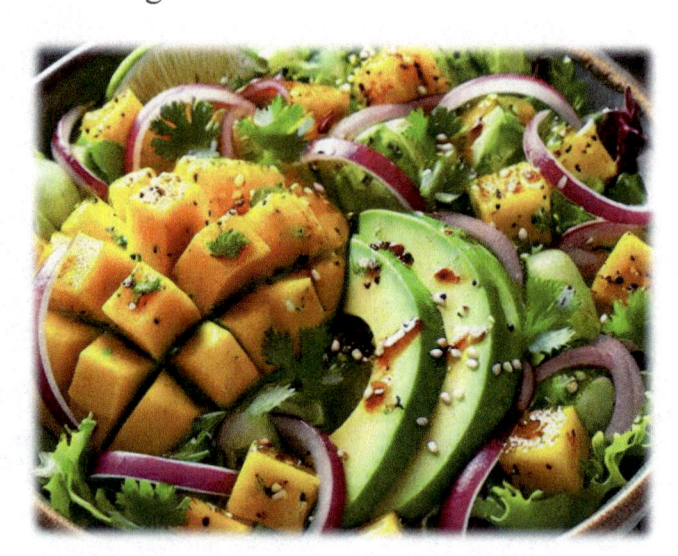

Cooking Time: 25 minutes

Instructions:

1. Heat olive oil in a pot over medium heat. Sauté onion and garlic until softened.
2. Add chickpeas, coconut milk, tomatoes, curry powder, salt, and pepper.
3. Simmer for 20 minutes.

15. Vegan Stuffed Portobello Mushrooms with Spinach and Almonds

Ingredients:

- 2 large portobello mushrooms, stems removed
- 1 cup fresh spinach, chopped
- 1 tbsp slivered almonds
- 1 clove garlic, minced
- 1 tsp olive oil
- Salt and pepper to taste

Cooking Time: 25 minutes

Instructions:

1. Preheat oven to 375°F (190°C).
2. Heat olive oil in a skillet. Sauté garlic and spinach until wilted.
3. Stuff mushrooms with spinach mixture and top with almonds.
4. Bake for 15-20 minutes.

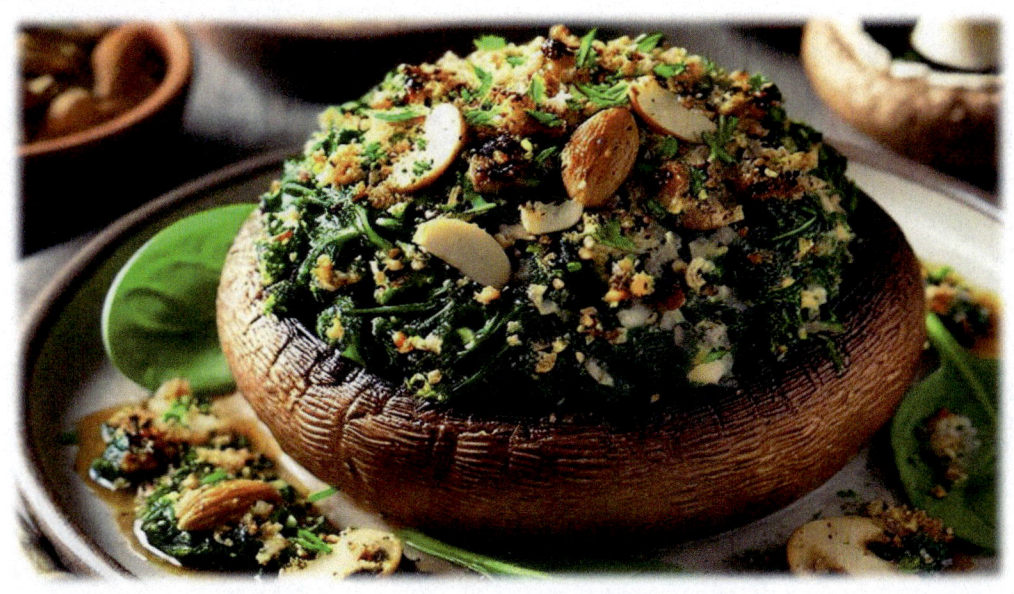

LUNCH IDEAS

1. Grilled Chicken & Quinoa Salad with Lemon Vinaigrette

Ingredients:

- 4 oz grilled chicken breast, sliced
- 1/2 cup cooked quinoa
- 2 cups mixed greens
- 1/4 cup cherry tomatoes, halved
- 1/4 cup cucumber, diced
- 1 tbsp lemon juice
- 1 tsp olive oil
- Salt and pepper to taste

Cooking Time: 20 minutes

Instructions:

1. Combine quinoa, mixed greens, tomatoes, and cucumber in a bowl.
2. Top with grilled chicken.
3. Whisk lemon juice, olive oil, salt, and pepper. Drizzle over the salad.

2. Veggie and Black Bean Burrito Bowl

Ingredients:

- 1/2 cup cooked brown rice
- 1/2 cup black beans, drained and rinsed
- 1/4 cup diced tomatoes
- 1/4 cup corn kernels
- 1/4 cup shredded lettuce
- 1 tbsp salsa
- 1 tsp lime juice

Cooking Time: 10 minutes

Instructions:

1. Layer brown rice, black beans, tomatoes, corn, and lettuce in a bowl.
2. Top with salsa and a squeeze of lime juice.

3. Smart Chicken Caesar Salad Wrap

Ingredients:

- 4 oz grilled chicken breast, sliced
- 1 whole wheat tortilla (low SmartPoints)
- 2 cups romaine lettuce, chopped
- 1 tbsp light Caesar dressing
- 1 tbsp grated Parmesan cheese

Cooking Time: 10 minutes

Instructions:

1. Spread Caesar dressing on the tortilla.
2. Layer lettuce, chicken, and Parmesan cheese.
3. Roll up the tortilla and serve.

4. Zucchini Noodles with Turkey Meatballs

Ingredients:

- 2 cups zucchini noodles (zoodles)
- 4 oz lean turkey meatballs
- 1/2 cup marinara sauce
- 1 tsp olive oil
- 1 clove garlic, minced

Cooking Time: 20 minutes

Instructions:

1. Heat olive oil in a skillet. Sauté garlic until fragrant.
2. Add turkey meatballs and cook until heated through.
3. Add marinara sauce and simmer for 5 minutes.
4. Serve over zucchini noodles.

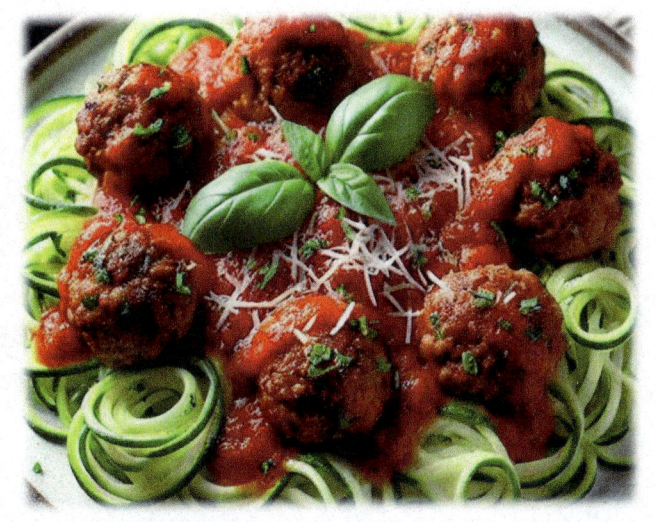

5. Crispy Chickpea Salad with Avocado

Ingredients:

- 1/2 cup chickpeas, drained and rinsed
- 1/2 avocado, diced
- 2 cups mixed greens
- 1 tbsp lemon juice
- 1 tsp olive oil
- Salt and pepper to taste

Cooking Time: 15 minutes

Instructions:

1. Toss chickpeas with olive oil, salt, and pepper. Roast at 400°F (200°C) for 10 minutes until crispy.
2. Combine mixed greens and avocado in a bowl.
3. Top with crispy chickpeas and drizzle with lemon juice.

6. Lemon Herb Grilled Salmon with Asparagus

Ingredients:

- 4 oz salmon fillet
- 1 cup asparagus spears
- 1 tbsp lemon juice
- 1 tsp olive oil
- 1/2 tsp dried thyme
- Salt and pepper to taste

Cooking Time: 15 minutes

Instructions:

1. Preheat grill or grill pan. Brush salmon and asparagus with olive oil and lemon juice.
2. Season with thyme, salt, and pepper.
3. Grill salmon for 4-5 minutes per side and asparagus for 5-7 minutes.

7. Spinach and Feta Stuffed Chicken Breast

Ingredients:

- 4 oz chicken breast
- 1/4 cup fresh spinach, chopped
- 1 tbsp crumbled feta cheese
- 1 tsp olive oil
- Salt and pepper to taste

Cooking Time: 25 minutes

Instructions:

1. Preheat oven to 375°F (190°C).
2. Cut a pocket into the chicken breast and stuff with spinach and feta.
3. Season with salt and pepper. Bake for 20-25 minutes until cooked through.

8. Tuna Salad Lettuce Wraps

Ingredients:

- 1 can (5 oz) tuna in water, drained
- 1 tbsp non-fat Greek yogurt
- 1 tsp Dijon mustard
- 1/4 cup diced celery
- 2 large lettuce leaves

Cooking Time: 10 minutes

Instructions:

1. Mix tuna, yogurt, mustard, and celery in a bowl.
2. Spoon mixture into lettuce leaves and wrap.

9. Mediterranean Chickpea Salad with Tzatziki

Ingredients:

- 1/2 cup chickpeas, drained and rinsed
- 1/4 cup cucumber, diced

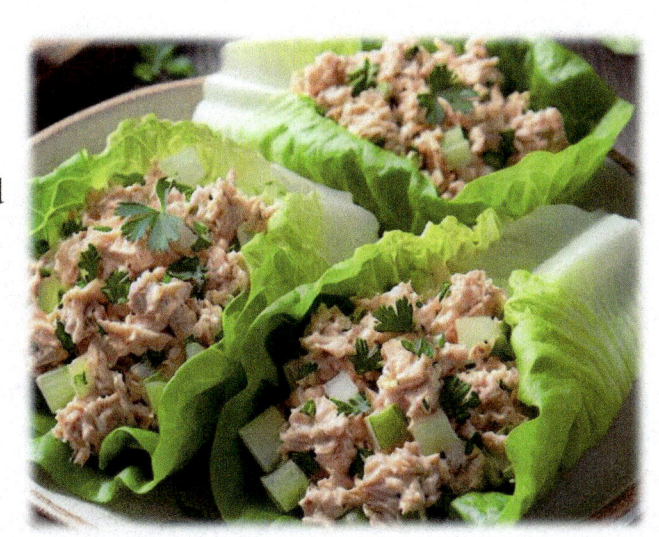

67 | *WEIGHT WATCHING* **SMARTPOINTS**

- 1/4 cup cherry tomatoes, halved
- 1/4 cup red onion, diced
- 2 tbsp tzatziki sauce (low SmartPoints)

Cooking Time: 10 minutes

Instructions:

1. Combine chickpeas, cucumber, tomatoes, and red onion in a bowl.
2. Top with tzatziki sauce.

10. Sweet Potato and Lentil Curry

Ingredients:

- 1 small sweet potato, peeled and diced
- 1/2 cup cooked lentils
- 1/2 cup light coconut milk
- 1/4 cup diced tomatoes
- 1/4 cup diced onion
- 1 clove garlic, minced
- 1 tsp olive oil
- 1/2 tsp curry powder
- Salt and pepper to taste

Cooking Time: 30 minutes

Instructions:

1. Heat olive oil in a pot. Sauté onion and garlic until softened.
2. Add sweet potato, lentils, coconut milk, tomatoes, curry powder, salt, and pepper.
3. Simmer for 20-25 minutes until sweet potatoes are tender.

11. Cabbage Stir-Fry with Shrimp and Garlic

Ingredients:

- 4 oz shrimp, peeled and deveined
- 2 cups shredded cabbage
- 1 clove garlic, minced
- 1 tsp olive oil

68 | *WEIGHT WATCHING* SMARTPOINTS

- 1 tbsp low-sodium soy sauce

Cooking Time: 15 minutes

Instructions:

1. Heat olive oil in a skillet. Sauté garlic until fragrant.
2. Add shrimp and cook until pink, about 3-4 minutes.
3. Add cabbage and soy sauce. Stir-fry for 5-7 minutes until tender.

12. Cauliflower Rice Stir Fry with Veggies and Tofu

Ingredients:

- 1 cup cauliflower rice
- 4 oz firm tofu, cubed
- 1/2 cup mixed vegetables (e.g., bell peppers, broccoli, snap peas)
- 1 tbsp low-sodium soy sauce
- 1 tsp olive oil

Cooking Time: 20 minutes

Instructions:

1. Heat olive oil in a skillet. Sauté tofu until golden, about 5 minutes.
2. Add vegetables and stir-fry for 5-7 minutes.
3. Add cauliflower rice and soy sauce. Cook for 3-4 minutes.

13. Turkey and Veggie Lettuce Wraps with Avocado

Ingredients:

- 4 oz ground turkey, cooked
- 1/4 cup diced bell peppers
- 1/4 cup shredded carrots
- 1/4 avocado, diced
- 2 large lettuce leaves

Cooking Time: 15 minutes

Instructions:

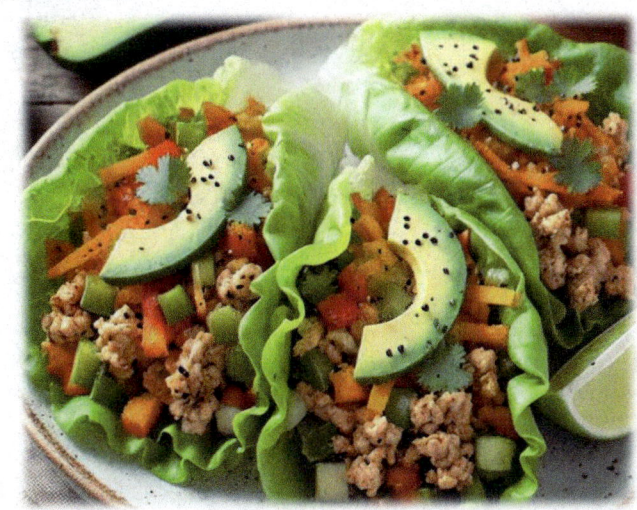

1. Cook ground turkey in a skillet until browned.
2. Layer turkey, bell peppers, carrots, and avocado on lettuce leaves.
3. Wrap and serve.

14. Roasted Veggie Buddha Bowl with Tahini Dressing

Ingredients:

- 1 cup roasted vegetables (e.g., zucchini, bell peppers, carrots)
- 1/2 cup cooked quinoa
- 1 tbsp tahini
- 1 tbsp lemon juice
- 1 tsp olive oil
- Salt and pepper to taste

Cooking Time: 30 minutes

Instructions:

1. Roast vegetables at 400°F (200°C) for 20 minutes.
2. Assemble roasted vegetables and quinoa in a bowl.
3. Whisk tahini, lemon juice, olive oil, salt, and pepper. Drizzle over the bowl.

15. Grilled Portobello Mushroom Burger with Spinach

Ingredients:

- 1 large portobello mushroom
- 1 whole wheat bun
- 1/2 cup fresh spinach
- 1 tsp olive oil
- 1 tsp balsamic vinegar

Cooking Time: 15 minutes

Instructions:

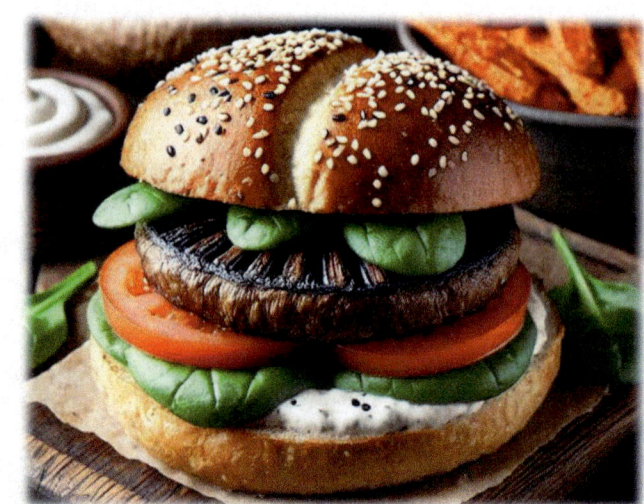

1. Preheat grill or grill pan. Brush mushroom with olive oil and balsamic vinegar.
2. Grill for 4-5 minutes per side.
3. Assemble the burger with spinach and grilled mushroom.

DELICIOUS DESSERTS

1. Chocolate-Dipped Strawberries with Almond Crunch

Ingredients:

- 6 large strawberries
- 1 oz dark chocolate (70% or higher), melted
- 1 tbsp crushed almonds

Cooking Time: 15 minutes

Instructions:

1. Dip strawberries in melted dark chocolate.
2. Sprinkle with crushed almonds.
3. Place on parchment paper and refrigerate until set.

2. Berry Coconut Chia Pudding Cups

Ingredients:

- 1/4 cup chia seeds
- 1 cup unsweetened almond milk
- 1/2 cup mixed berries
- 1 tsp honey or sugar-free syrup

Cooking Time: Overnight (5 minutes prep)

Instructions:

1. Mix chia seeds and almond milk in a jar. Refrigerate overnight.
2. Layer chia pudding with berries in a cup. Drizzle with honey or syrup.

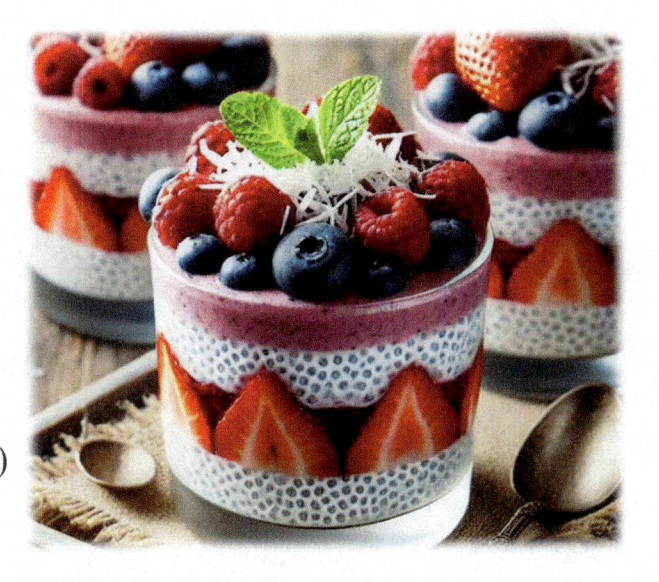

3. Skinny Apple Cinnamon Crumble

Ingredients:

- 1 apple, peeled and diced
- 1/4 cup oats
- 1 tsp cinnamon
- 1 tsp honey or sugar-free syrup
- 1 tsp olive oil

Cooking Time: 25 minutes

Instructions:

1. Preheat oven to 350°F (175°C).
2. Toss apple with cinnamon and honey. Place in a baking dish.
3. Mix oats with olive oil and sprinkle over the apples.
4. Bake for 20-25 minutes until golden.

4. Mini Cheesecake Bites with Fresh Berries

Ingredients:

- 4 oz low-fat cream cheese
- 1/4 cup non-fat Greek yogurt
- 1 tsp honey or sugar-free syrup
- 1/4 cup fresh berries

Cooking Time: 10 minutes

Instructions:

1. Mix cream cheese, yogurt, and honey until smooth.
2. Spoon into small cups and top with fresh berries.

5. Sugar-Free Chocolate Mousse

Ingredients:

- 1 ripe avocado
- 2 tbsp unsweetened cocoa powder

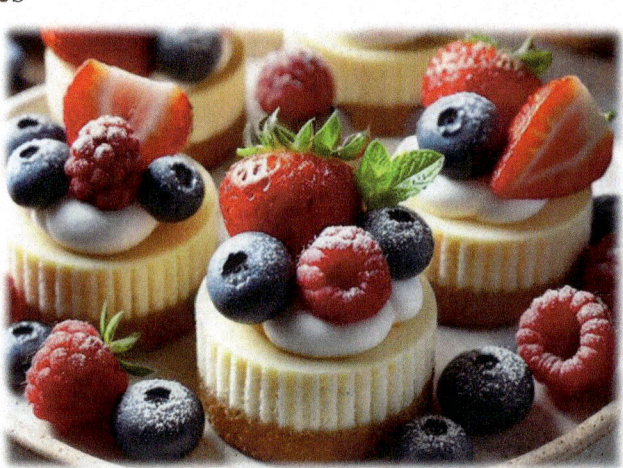

- 1 tbsp honey or sugar-free syrup
- 1/4 tsp vanilla extract

Cooking Time: 10 minutes

Instructions:

1. Blend avocado, cocoa powder, honey, and vanilla in a food processor until smooth.
2. Chill for 1 hour before serving.

6. Peanut Butter Banana Ice Cream Bites

Ingredients:

- 1 ripe banana, sliced
- 1 tbsp natural peanut butter

Cooking Time: 2 hours (freezing time)

Instructions:

1. Spread peanut butter between banana slices to make sandwiches.
2. Freeze for 2 hours until firm.

7. Lemon Yogurt Pound Cake

Ingredients:

- 1/2 cup almond flour
- 1/4 cup non-fat Greek yogurt
- 1 egg
- 1 tbsp lemon juice
- 1 tsp lemon zest
- 1 tsp honey or sugar-free syrup

Cooking Time: 30 minutes

Instructions:

1. Preheat oven to 350°F (175°C).
2. Mix almond flour, yogurt, egg, lemon juice, lemon zest, and honey.

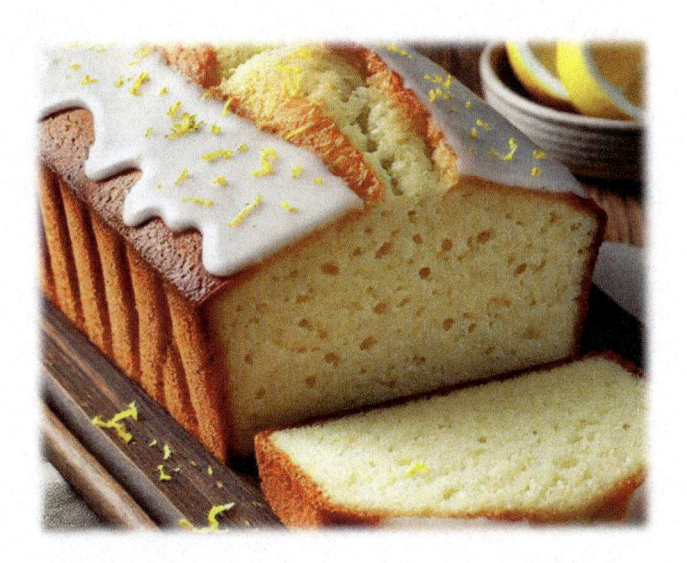

3. Pour into a greased loaf pan and bake for 25-30 minutes.

8. SmartPoints-Friendly Chocolate Avocado Pudding

Ingredients:

- 1 ripe avocado
- 2 tbsp unsweetened cocoa powder
- 1 tbsp honey or sugar-free syrup
- 1/4 tsp vanilla extract

Cooking Time: 10 minutes

Instructions:

1. Blend avocado, cocoa powder, honey, and vanilla in a food processor until smooth.
2. Chill for 1 hour before serving.

9. Coconut-Almond Energy Bites

Ingredients:

- 1/4 cup oats
- 1 tbsp almond butter
- 1 tbsp shredded coconut
- 1 tsp honey or sugar-free syrup

Cooking Time: 10 minutes

Instructions:

1. Mix oats, almond butter, coconut, and honey in a bowl.
2. Roll into small balls and refrigerate until firm.

10. No-Bake Protein-Packed Chocolate Bars

Ingredients:

- 1/4 cup oats
- 1 scoop chocolate protein powder
- 1 tbsp almond butter

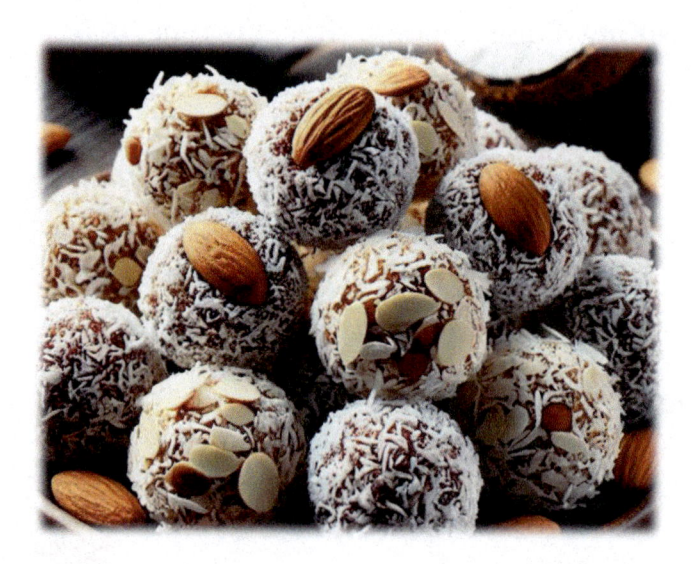

- 1 tsp honey or sugar-free syrup

Cooking Time: 10 minutes

Instructions:

1. Mix oats, protein powder, almond butter, and honey in a bowl.
2. Press into a small dish and refrigerate until firm. Cut into bars.

11. Cinnamon-Spiced Baked Pears with Walnuts

Ingredients:

- 1 pear, halved and cored
- 1/2 tsp cinnamon
- 1 tbsp chopped walnuts
- 1 tsp honey or sugar-free syrup

Cooking Time: 25 minutes

Instructions:

1. Preheat oven to 350°F (175°C).
2. Place pear halves on a baking dish. Sprinkle with cinnamon and walnuts.
3. Drizzle with honey and bake for 20-25 minutes.

12. Healthy Fruit Sorbet Popsicles

Ingredients:

- 1 cup mixed berries
- 1/2 cup unsweetened almond milk
- 1 tsp honey or sugar-free syrup

Cooking Time: 4 hours (freezing time)

Instructions:

1. Blend berries, almond milk, and honey until smooth.
2. Pour into popsicle molds and freeze for 4 hours.

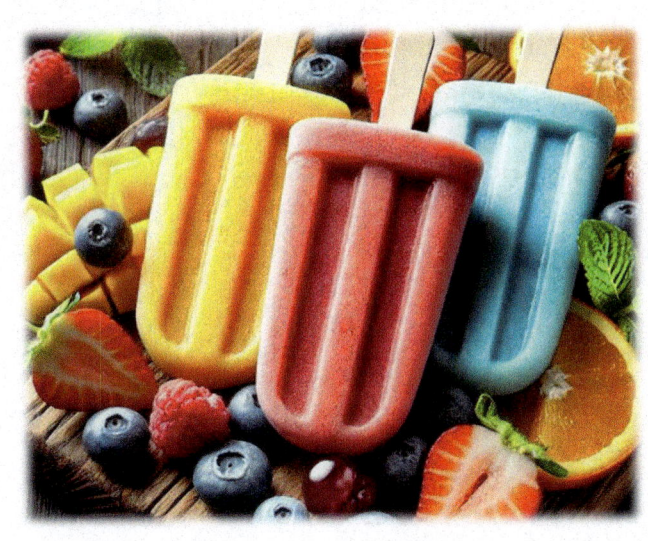

13. Almond Flour Chocolate Chip Cookies

Ingredients:

- 1/2 cup almond flour
- 1 tbsp honey or sugar-free syrup
- 1 tbsp dark chocolate chips
- 1/4 tsp vanilla extract

Cooking Time: 15 minutes

Instructions:

1. Preheat oven to 350°F (175°C).
2. Mix almond flour, honey, chocolate chips, and vanilla.
3. Drop spoonfuls onto a baking sheet and bake for 10-12 minutes.

14. Baked Cinnamon Apple Donuts

Ingredients:

- 1/2 cup almond flour
- 1/4 cup unsweetened applesauce
- 1/2 tsp cinnamon
- 1 tsp honey or sugar-free syrup

Cooking Time: 20 minutes

Instructions:

1. Preheat oven to 350°F (175°C).
2. Mix almond flour, applesauce, cinnamon, and honey.
3. Pour into a greased donut pan and bake for 15-18 minutes.

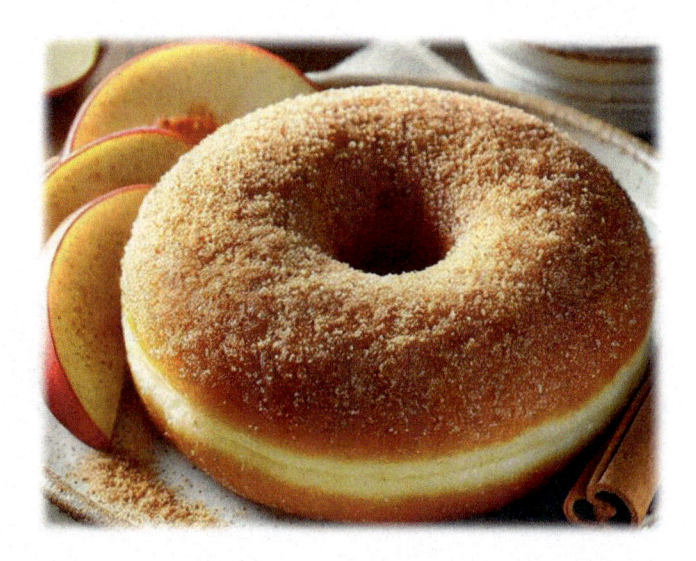

15. Sugar-Free Pumpkin Spice Muffins

Ingredients:

- 1/2 cup almond flour
- 1/4 cup pumpkin puree
- 1/2 tsp pumpkin spice
- 1 tsp honey or sugar-free syrup

Cooking Time: 20 minutes

Instructions:

1. Preheat oven to 350°F (175°C).
2. Mix almond flour, pumpkin puree, pumpkin spice, and honey.
3. Pour into a greased muffin tin and bake for 15-18 minutes.

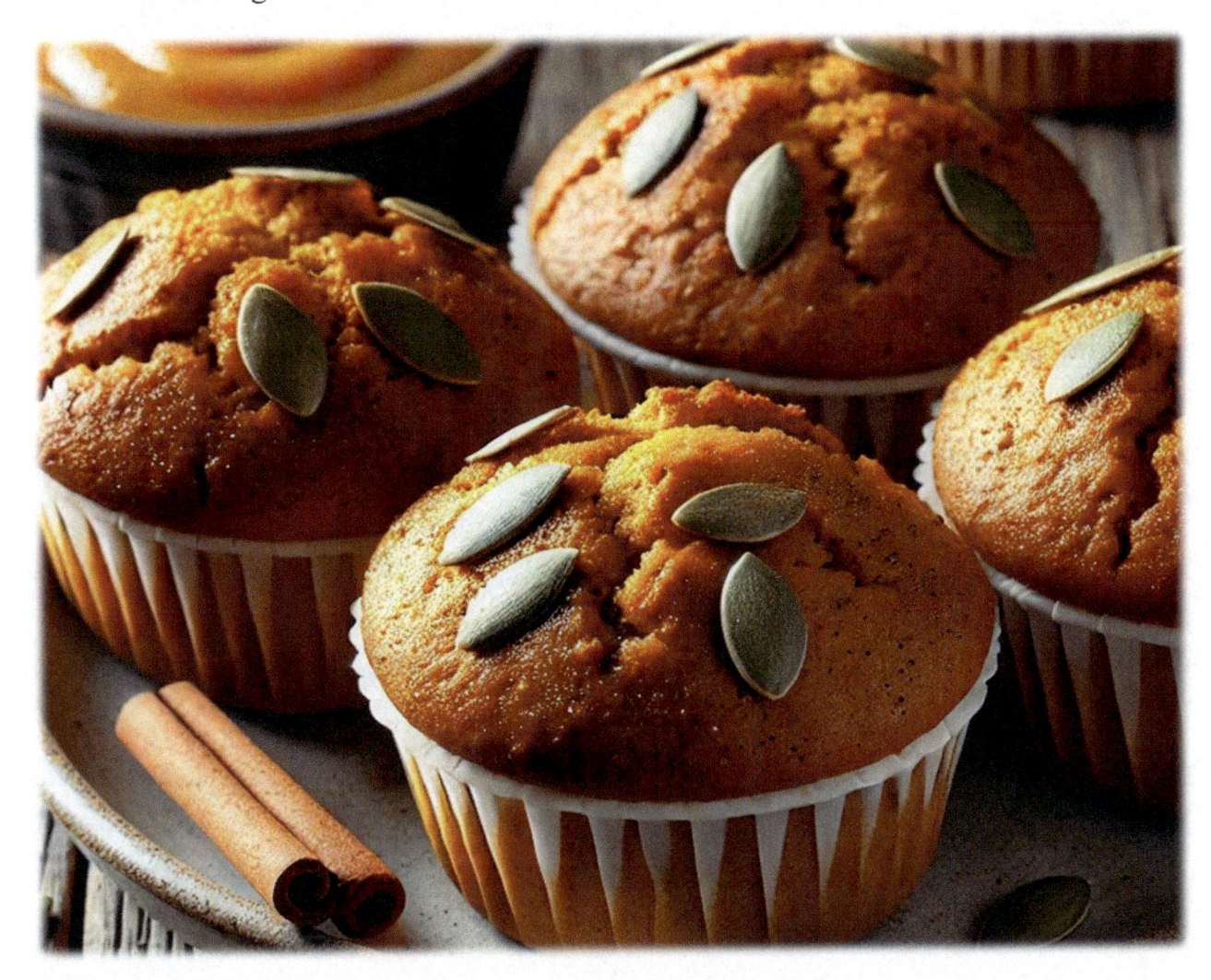

SMARTPOINTS COOKING TIPS AND TRICKS

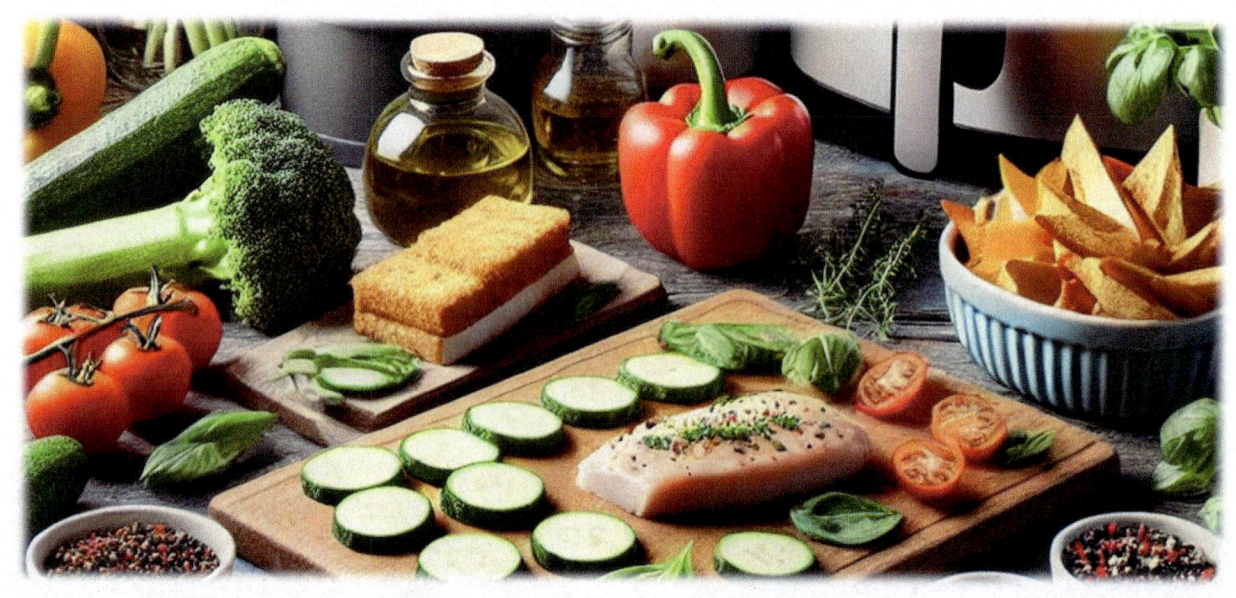

Cooking with SmartPoints: Tips for Success

The practice of preparing food with low SmartPoints does not force people to compromise the flavor of their meals. Follow these steps to prepare delicious healthy food along with nutritional aspects:

High-point sauces can be replaced with low-calorie flavors that come from using basil and cilantro and paprika or cumin spices.

Decline frying as a cooking method because you should use grill baking steaming or air-frying to reduce added fats in meals.

Dishes receive no extra points when you use lemon or lime juice to provide a fresh flavor profile.

Zero-point vegetables such as zucchini spinach and bell peppers should be used to increase the bulk of meals.

You should select lean protein options which include chicken breast turkey or tofu because they help maintain low point value and provide a prolonged feeling of fullness.

Recipe Examples:

- You can create a low-point grilled chicken main course by marinating chicken breast in garlic and lemon juice together with dried herbs before placing it on the grill.
- Veggie Stir-Fry: Sauté zucchini, bell peppers, and mushrooms with soy sauce and ginger for a quick, low-point meal.
- Air-Fryer Sweet Potato Fries require a lightweight coating of oil together with paprika before air-frying to create crispy low-point satisfaction for snack time.
- The tactics mentioned in this essay will help you prepare delicious foods within your assigned SmartPoints spending limit.

Simple Techniques to Lower Points Without Sacrificing Flavor

The act of lowering SmartPoints values does not require any compromises regarding culinary flavor. Try these simple techniques:

Ingredient Substitutions: Swap high-point ingredients for lower-point alternatives. Greek yogurt makes an ideal replacement for sour cream and zucchini noodles function as an excellent pasta substitute.

Portion sizes of high-point food should be limited while zero-point veggies should fill most of the plate.

Baking along with grilling and steaming give better results than frying because they minimize fat addition.

Adapted Dishes:

- To make pizza use a whole-wheat tortilla as the base and add tomato sauce with veggies while calling for a minimal amount of low-fat cheese.
- The dish maintains its satisfaction by incorporating half the pasta with spiralized zucchini which reduces points.
- Dessert: Make a fruit salad with a drizzle of honey instead of a high-point cake.
- Very slight modifications in your food preparation methods will significantly reduce your SmartPoint count.

EMBRACING A SUSTAINABLE WW LIFESTYLE

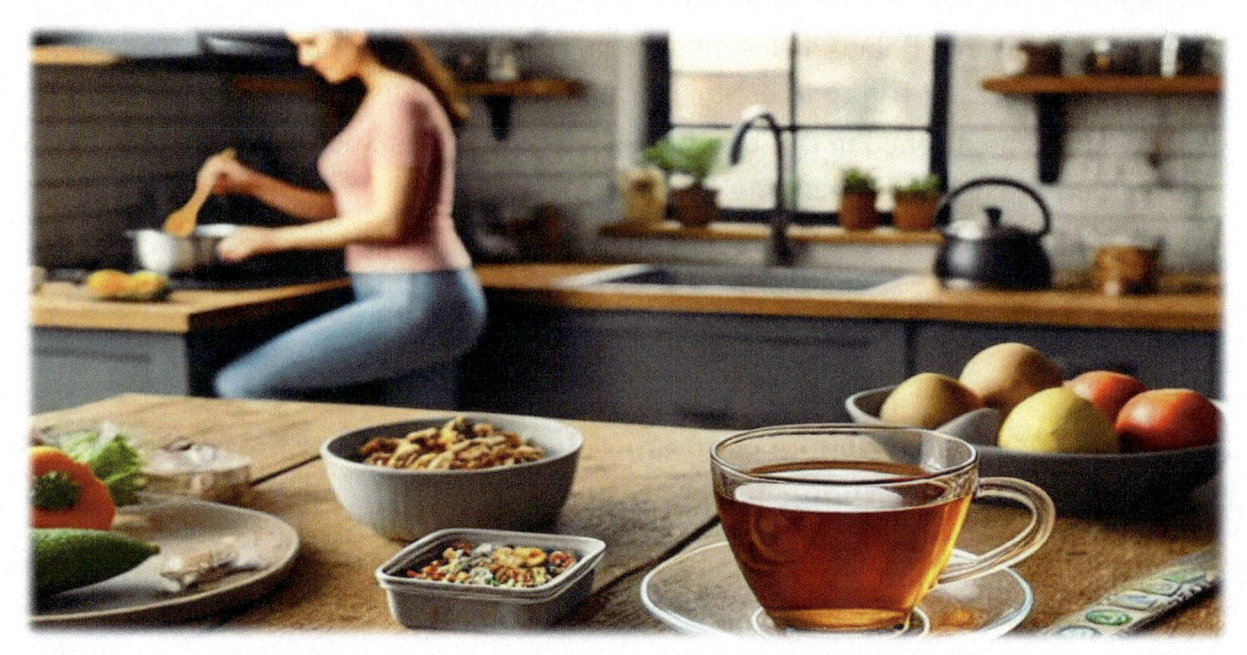

Making WW a Part of Your Everyday Life

Getting on a system with WW SmartPoints is the key to long-term success. To have it become a part of your life and you, here is what to do:

- Begin with one habit: See tracking what time you go to bed or planning dinners for the next 7 days.
- Be Consistent: Utilize the WW application to track dinners every day, no materialistic events or weekends.
- Way To Overcome Challenges: If you cross your SmartPoints graph, do not freak out—simply return to your routine the accompanying day.
- Routines: (COMIDAS1) concocts meals First Off, has good Responsibility ON call, and creates a meal, plan follows weekly for routine organization.
- For example, Ana, a hectic mother, began by monitoring her breakfast, and steadily missed lunch, and dinner. Sporadically, she naturally fell into lower point menus and more so in tune with her eating.
- Making small, regular changes helps you permanently turn SmartPoints into a healthy and sustainable lifestyle for your health and wellness goals.

Practical Strategies for Long-Term Health and Well-being

WW SmartPoints System functions beyond dietary restrictions as it provides permanent health management tools. WW SmartPoints System can achieve long-term success through the following methods:

Maintain your favorite foods by eating them sparingly and center your diet on nutritious foods that have low SmartPoint numbers.

Make sleep along with hydration and effective stress management your number one priority since they promote entire body wellness.

To achieve better results than flawless outcomes set achievable everyday objectives. Recognize your achievements through daily achievements including following your budget or cooking fresh recipes.

Pair SmartPoints with physical exercise because this approach will increase your energy levels alongside maintaining weight loss results.

John a WW member enjoyed pizza as one of his favorite foods by eating a piece which was 12 SmartPoints combined with a big salad which earned zero SmartPoints. Through practice, he developed the ability to create nutritious versions at home by substituting whole wheat crust and adding vegetables.

Your progress will stay steady and your lifestyle will become both healthier and happier by setting practical objectives and prioritizing equilibrium with self-help practices.

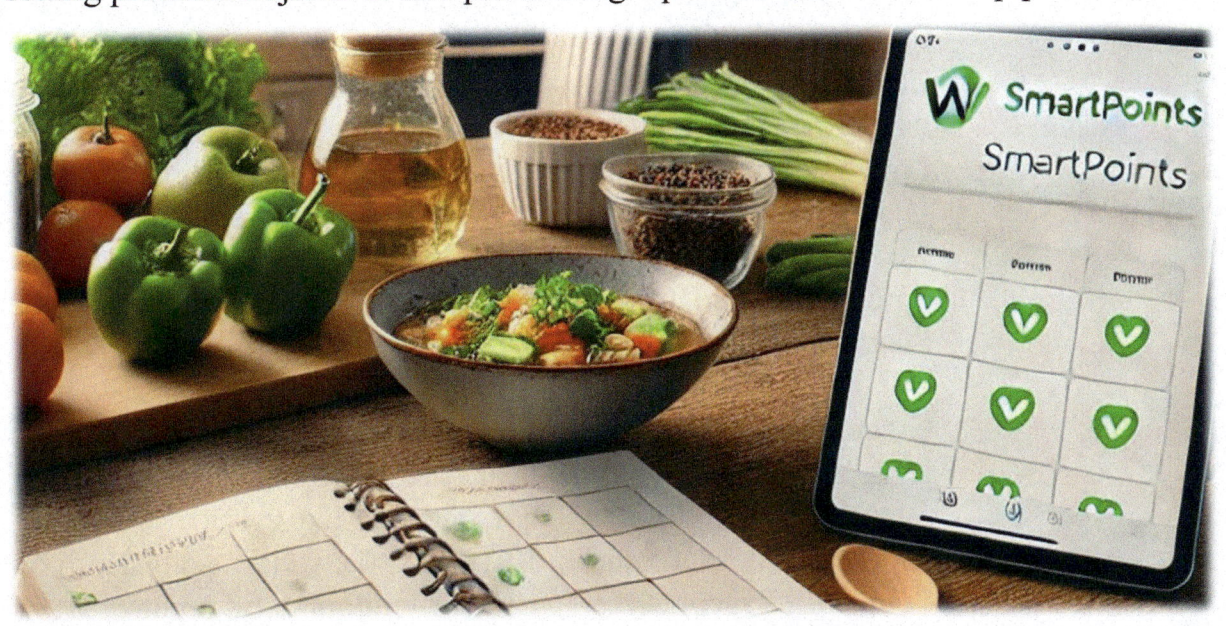

BONUS: 30-DAY MEAL PLAN

Category	Meal Ideas	SmartPoints-Friendly Tip
BREAKFAST DELIGHTS	Spinach & Mushroom Scramble with Feta	Use egg whites to reduce points while keeping protein high.
	Berry Almond Butter Smoothie	Use unsweetened almond milk and a small portion of almond butter for lower points.
	Oatmeal with Fresh Fruit and Cinnamon	Add zero-point fruits like berries or sliced bananas for natural sweetness.
	Avocado, Tomato & Egg Breakfast Bowl	Use half an avocado to keep points low while enjoying healthy fats.
	Coconut Yogurt with Mango and Chia Seeds	Opt for unsweetened coconut yogurt and fresh mango to minimize added sugars.
SATISFYING SNACKS	Spicy Baked Sweet Potato Wedges	Skip the oil and use a light spray for crispiness without extra points.
	Crunchy Veggie Spring Rolls with Peanut Dipping Sauce	Use rice paper wraps and a small amount of peanut sauce for flavor.
	Crispy Baked Edamame with Sea Salt	A high-protein, low-point snack that's perfect for munching.
	Zesty Guacamole with Baked Veggie Chips	Use cucumber or zucchini slices as dippers for zero-point crunch.
	Cauliflower Buffalo Bites with Blue Cheese Dip	Bake instead of frying to keep points low.
HEARTY SOUPS & STEWS	Low-calorie chicken and Vegetable Soup	Use skinless chicken breast and load up on zero-point veggies like celery and carrots.
	Spicy Lentil and Tomato Stew	Lentils are high in protein and fiber, making this stew filling and low in points.
	Creamy Cauliflower and Leek Soup	Blend cauliflower for creaminess without adding high-point ingredients like cream.
	Roasted Butternut Squash Soup with Sage	Roasting the squash adds depth of flavor without extra points.

	Turkey and Kale White Bean Soup	Use lean ground turkey and plenty of kale for a nutrient-packed meal.
FLAVORFUL SALADS	Greek Salad with Grilled Chicken and Feta	Use a light olive oil and lemon dressing to keep points low.
	Avocado and Black Bean Salad with Lime Vinaigrette	Add corn and cherry tomatoes for extra color and flavor.
	Roasted Beet Salad with Arugula and Goat Cheese	Use a small amount of goat cheese for flavor without too many points.
	Apple, Walnut, and Spinach Salad with Balsamic Glaze	Measure walnuts to control portion size and points.
	Chopped Chickpea Salad with Cucumber and Red Onion	Chickpeas are a great low-point source of protein and fiber.
SEAFOOD	Grilled Lemon Herb Salmon	Salmon is rich in omega-3s and low in points when grilled.
	Crispy Baked Fish Tacos with Avocado Slaw	Use corn tortillas and load up on avocado slaw for flavor.
	Smart Shrimp Scampi with Zoodles	Swap pasta for zucchini noodles to save points.
	Spicy Sriracha Tuna Poke Bowl	Use brown rice and plenty of veggies for a filling, low-point meal.
	Garlic Butter Shrimp & Asparagus	Use a small amount of light butter or olive oil for flavor.
PLANT-BASED OPTIONS	Quinoa & Black Bean Stuffed Sweet Potatoes	Sweet potatoes are zero points and pair perfectly with quinoa and beans.
	Lentil and Veggie Buddha Bowl	Add a variety of roasted veggies for texture and flavor.
	Chickpea Salad with Lemon Tahini Dressing	Use a light tahini dressing to keep points low.
	Spaghetti Squash with Roasted Tomato and Pesto	Spaghetti squash is a zero-point alternative to pasta.
	Cauliflower and Chickpea Tacos with Avocado Salsa	Use lettuce wraps instead of tortillas to save points.
LUNCH IDEAS	Grilled Chicken & Quinoa Salad with Lemon Vinaigrette	Use a light vinaigrette and plenty of fresh herbs for flavor.

	Veggie and Black Bean Burrito Bowl	Skip the rice and add extra veggies to keep points low.
	Smart Chicken Caesar Salad Wrap	Use a whole-wheat wrap and light Caesar dressing.
	Zucchini Noodles with Turkey Meatballs	Use lean turkey and zucchini noodles for a low-point, high-protein meal.
	Crispy Chickpea Salad with Avocado	Add a squeeze of lime for extra zing without adding points.
DELICIOUS DESSERTS	Chocolate-Dipped Strawberries with Almond Crunch	Use dark chocolate and a small amount of crushed almonds for a low-point treat.
	Berry Coconut Chia Pudding Cups	Use unsweetened coconut milk and fresh berries for natural sweetness.
	Skinny Apple Cinnamon Crumble	Use oats and a touch of cinnamon for a low-point crumble topping.
	Mini Cheesecake Bites with Fresh Berries	Use light cream cheese and a small portion of graham cracker crumbs.
	Sugar-Free Chocolate Mousse	Use unsweetened cocoa powder and a sugar substitute for a guilt-free dessert.

Tips for Success

TIP	DESCRIPTION	WHY IT HELPS
MEAL PREP	Spend a few hours on the weekend prepping ingredients or cooking meals for the week.	Saves time during busy weekdays and ensures you have healthy, SmartPoints-friendly meals ready.
PORTION CONTROL	Use measuring cups, spoons, or a food scale to stay within your SmartPoints budget.	Helps you avoid overeating and stay on track with your daily SmartPoints allowance.
STAY HYDRATED	Drink plenty of water throughout the day to stay full and energized.	Keeps you hydrated, reduces cravings, and supports overall health.
TRACK EVERYTHING	Use the WW app to log meals, snacks, and drinks to stay accountable.	Keeps you aware of your SmartPoints usage and helps you make mindful choices.

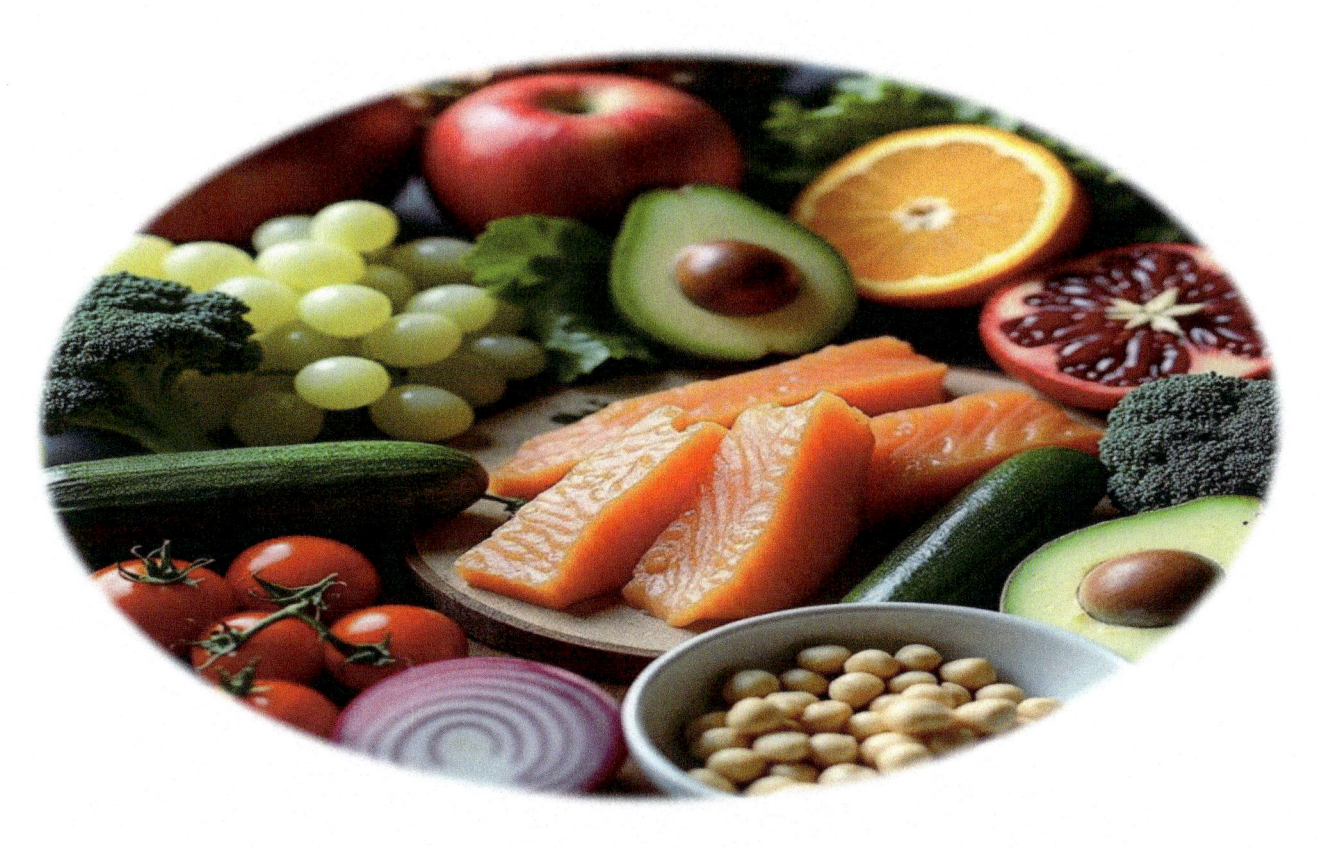

"Thank you for Being Part of The WEIGHT-WATCHING SMARTPOINTS Journey"

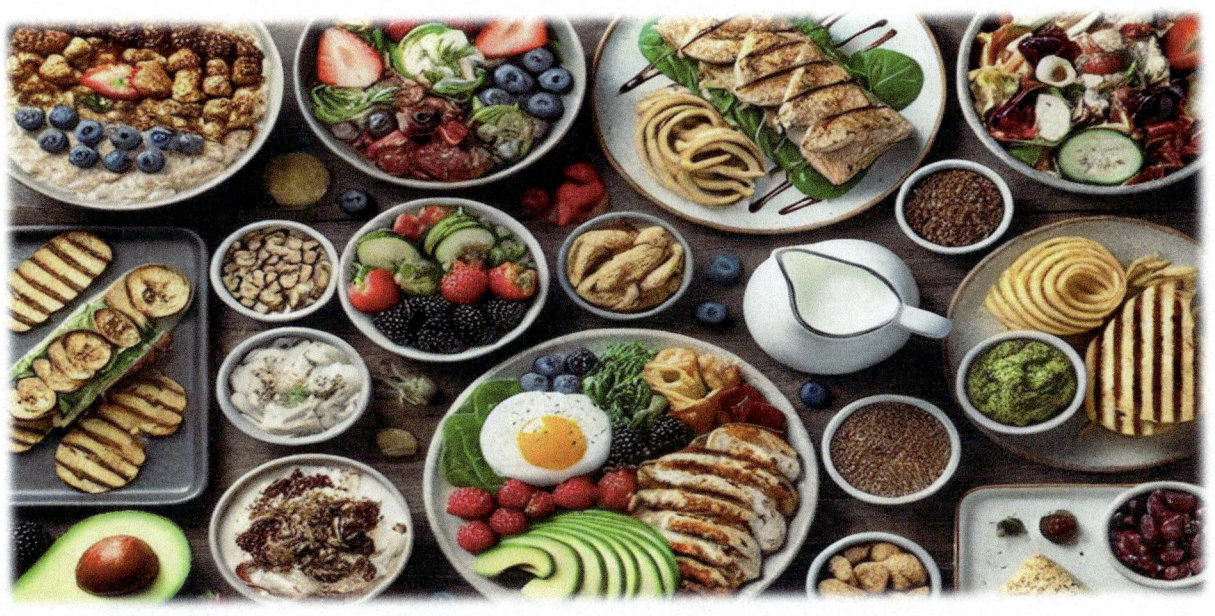

85 | *WEIGHT WATCHING* **SMARTPOINTS**

Printed in Great Britain
by Amazon